The Lost Kitchen: Reflections and Recipes from an Alzheimer's Caregiver is an honest and heartfelt look at the hidden gifts of living with a parent with Alzheimer's. Miriam Green weaves poetry, recipes and anecdotes into a nourishing whole as she details her family's struggle to maintain balance—and laughter—in the face of her mother's diagnosis and deterioration. Throughout this most personal of stories, Naomi has been Miriam's greatest teacher. Together, they remind us how to love and laugh in a world that is often confusing and painful.

KUDOS for *The Lost Kitchen*

"In page after page of *The Lost Kitchen*, we learn from Miriam Green's example how to be a loving and responsible daughter. The wisdom of her words and the compassion, understanding and even humor in her responses to her mother's illness teach us what it means to navigate the struggle and remain buoyed up by one's own resources."
~ Linda Stern Zisquit, *Ritual Bath*

"This book is wonderful. It has a unique style that I have never met before. And a strange technique where making food and poetry, and the mother's desperation are all in the soup together. So we get the joys of desire and the crying of family love woven together in a happy mix. It comes alive and speaks to you directly. You awake and sing and cry all at once."
~ Bernard Kops, *The Hamlet of Stepney Green*

"A moving and inspirational story of memories – past and present, lost and found – set in and around the kitchen table. This book is certain to bring comfort to anyone struggling with aging parents or coping with loss, strengthening your courage and reaffirming your faith even during life's most difficult moments."
~ Tamar Genger MA, RD, Kosher Network International

ACKNOWLEDGMENTS

This book has been in the making for more than a few years. It has taken many turns, growing ever larger as my experiences caring for my mom piled up and began to sort themselves into categories and chapters. Early readers included Reesa Stone, Drora Gopas, and Chanah Rubin, who encouraged me to continue. Judy Spanglet was there in the beginning with support and advice. And Yael Unterman came later and whipped me into shape.

My father, Jack, now cooks more than omelets. Together with my mom, he nurtured me with a sense that I could accomplish anything.

My little brother did a good job of annoying me when we were young. These days, he is my confidant. Simon is intimately on this journey with us, though he is thousands of miles away. He is part of our daily conversations with Mom. So, too, Sharon and Shoshana. Sharon brought to life this book's cover in style and dedication.

During my parents' many visits to our house, the highlight was always taking Mom with me to synagogue to hear her clear soprano rising in prayer. I want to thank our wonderful community for accepting my mom with all the difficulties that Alzheimer's brings, and for treating her with true kindness and love.

My fellow poets helped sharpen and clarify my poetic voice. And my recipe testers added flavor to this book.

Finally, my little band of Greens: I look forward to growing old together (because we aren't there yet) with my husband Jeff in love and partnership. And Rafi, Hadas, Liora, Hillel, and Roi have filled my life with blessings and light.

The Lost Kitchen

Reflections and Recipes from
an Alzheimer's Caregiver

Miriam Green

A Black Opal Books Publication

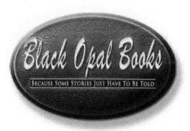

GENRE: NON-FICTION/SELF-HELP

This book is a work of non-fiction. All information and opinions expressed herein are the views of the author. This publication is intended to provide accurate and authoritative information concerning the subject matter covered and is for informational purposes only. Neither the author nor the publisher is attempting to provide legal or medical advice/diagnosis of any kind. All trademarks, service marks, registered trademarks, and registered service marks are the property of their respective owners and if used herein are for identification purposes only. The publisher does not have any control over or assume any responsibility for author or third-party websites or their contents.

DEDICATION

To my mom, Naomi Cohen,
who, even in her advanced stage of Alzheimer's,
remains my most stalwart teacher
of love and compassion.

"On the housewife's shoulders rests the responsibility of providing nourishing and appetizing meals for her family."

~ Florence Greenberg, *Jewish Cookery Book*

Equilibrium is simply
that moment when the present
is as real as the past
or the future, when the air
that nourishes us
we breathe
without thinking.

~ Linda Pastan, "Balance," *Heroes in Disguise*

Table of Contents

Brain Tangles

Dandelions
clump like tumors
in the riotous garden

of your mind. Empty diagnosis,
you insist. No one tells
the truth, not the doctors,

not your husband. Not God
behind His one-way mirrors. Sometimes
you admit you're confused.

The clock's hands read
like a foreign language.
House plants wither without

water. There's a book in the freezer,
coins in the sugar bowl.
You jam the wrong key

into the locked door and
rage when it won't open.
You wander rooms

you have already abandoned.
If there is a key, it is hidden
in the chaos of your drawers.

We sort through piles
of single socks and match
the pairs as if

we could patch your brain,
tangles that constrict
all knowledge

until even your name is lost.

FOREWORD

I'm not a foodie. I don't have a zealous interest in food, I don't gawk at expensive and obscure ingredients in grocery stores, and I don't own a fancy food processor or a meat thermometer or even a scale. What I do have is a desire to cook practically and simply. Cooking meals for my family is one way to express my love for them. When I make something they love to eat, they taste my love in the food, and, I'm pleased to say, they thank me for it. I remember how proud I felt when my young kids, aged nine, six, and four, unanimously voted quiche as their favorite dish. Not even pizza from the pizza parlor could unsettle that choice.

After twenty-five years of marriage, the recipe for quiche is one I know by heart. However, the first time I attempt a new dish, I invariably follow a recipe. Only after I've made it several times do I add signature changes to personalize it. I learned that from my mom, Naomi Cohen. Mom was a formidable housewife and an excellent cook. She inducted me into a practical cooking life. I watched as she bought and salted meat in our sink before turning it into delicious roast; as she cut and chopped vegetables for soup; or even as she made me sandwiches for school. Tasked with making my own sandwiches when I turned twelve, I toasted slices of round dark bread and layered them with cheese, avocado, tomato, sprouts, and a generous helping of mayonnaise. To me, each sandwich was an act of creation.

When my mom developed Alzheimer's, her mounting mistakes in the kitchen encouraged my dad, Jack, to try his own hand at creating meals. As he moved from making omelets to fancier dishes, he finally began to understand how much Mom had given him throughout their many years of marriage. And as he sought my assistance in his newfound position of "chief cook and bottle washer," I realized I had a new cooking partner and another reason to see cooking as an essential element in my life.

This book is a combination of recipes, poetry, and prose about my family and how we have shared and confronted the demands of Mom's Alzheimer's. Mom's functioning deteriorated during the writing of this book, such that many things described in the present tense are now beyond her capabilities. Throughout this most personal of stories, Mom has been my greatest teacher. She has taught me how to love and laugh in a world that is often confusing and painful.

Mom has unknowingly encouraged me to give of myself and to express as best I can the advice I've learned about Alzheimer's. I hope that it can help others in our position who are caring for loved ones no longer in their prime but still loved, still wanted, and still needed.

𝒞𝒟𝒞𝒟

Why call this book *The Lost Kitchen?* One of the gifts of caring for someone with Alzheimer's is learning how to laugh through your tears. The kitchen is lost to Mom, but we can reclaim it by remembering with humor the life she once lived. Here's a version of a popular joke about Alzheimer's.

Joan and Stan are watching TV on the couch in the living room. Joan gets up.

"I'm going to the kitchen to get some ice cream. Do you want some?" she asks.

"Sure," says Stan. "I'd also like some strawberries on top. And sprinkles."

"Okay," says Joan. She starts to walk away.

"Are you going to remember that?" asks Stan. "Do you want to write it down?"

"I can remember that," says Joan, "I've still got half a brain."

Joan leaves and is gone for about twenty minutes. When she returns, her hands are empty.

"Where's my tea?" asks Stan.

"Where's the kitchen?" asks Joan.

Miriam Green
Israel, 2018

Recipe for a Small Star

for Ima

Ingredients:
2 cups sifted memories
½ tsp unfiltered light
1 Tbsp clarified passion
3 sun-dried hearts
Pinch of time

Directions:
Say her name. Say
her name. Shout it. Loud,
louder. Louder.
String the memories together
like beads of light
that explode in a brilliant flash
in the night sky.

INTRODUCTION

Those early months were difficult. I didn't want to believe the diagnosis. If I was being honest with myself, though, I knew with certainty that Mom had Alzheimer's.

I was not prepared for the disarray that Alzheimer's brought into our lives. I didn't realize the extent to which every emotion I displayed would be amplified in Mom's behavior. I couldn't grasp fully that Mom had entered an alternate reality where her unchecked and discordant emotions often burst out indiscriminately. I had to keep reminding myself that Mom was blameless, that it was the disease affecting her, that her tantrums and fear and gaping holes in her memory were out of her control.

The first thing I learned was that each person afflicted with Alzheimer's reacts differently to the disease. After she was diagnosed, Mom refused to entertain any notion of being ill. If my dad or I brought up the subject of Alzheimer's, she would say, "That has nothing to do with me!" and furiously walk away. I had heard that some Alzheimer's patients were not only aware of their situation but actively fought against it. This was not the case with Mom. After the third or fourth try, we decided that we would not discuss it with her.

There have been hard times: On more than one occasion, I have locked Mom in her own house when she frantically wanted to get out; I removed toothpaste from her hair when she used her toothbrush as a hairbrush; I helped her remove the two skirts and five pairs of underwear she'd donned; I caused her to panic when I missed her return to our restaurant table because I was foolishly playing with my phone. And amazing dividends: her radiant smile, her memory for music, and her snorting laughter at silly jokes.

It took a slow while, but eventually I found ways that helped us minimize the confusion. It had to start with my own behavior. It meant acknowledging Mom's reality, listening patiently to her often incoherent statements, bringing her into conversations instead of talking over her head, assuaging her anger, tamping down my own anger, finding ways to make her laugh, being in the moment, and loving her unconditionally. The effect was like shining a bright light in a dark place and finding that the room was filled with hidden blessings.

Mom did acknowledge her growing memory loss. More than once I held her as she cried in my arms at the utter confusion she felt, at her brain's inability to process the social and verbal cues all around her.

Sharing my pain and bewilderment with other people in the same situation helped. A friend, Judy, whose mother also had Alzheimer's, took me out for coffee and openly answered every question I put to her. I was affected most profoundly by Judy relating that her mom did not know who she was anymore. I could not then imagine how a child's whole life could be swallowed up by this disease.

Online sites with technical and scientific information were often overwhelming in their intensity, and I shied away from them. Books were better, as were websites with personal accounts. I could read at my own pace, absorbing facts and suggestions that pertained to our situation, finding solace in other caregiver's voices.

Ultimately, my own experiences taught me how to move forward while maintaining as normal a life as possible. We wanted to keep Mom involved and engaged in family celebrations, holidays, trips, and daily activities. She needed the stimulation and we needed that connection to her in all her roles—wife, mother, grandmother, sister, daughter.

I discovered how to use Mom's memory loss to my advantage, and how to calm her when she raged against us. I learned how damaging certain illnesses were for an Alzheimer's patient, and how important noninvasive blood and urine tests could be—if Mom could be convinced to comply. I found reserves of kindness and patience in myself that I didn't know I had and creativity that I used to keep her happy. I accepted the beauty of living in the moment and learned to give of myself whole-heartedly even as Mom forgot who I was. I became, in essence, my mother's mother.

e⁄ɔe⁄ɔ

The last few years have been filled with such surprising situations, many of which have tested me to my limits. Through it all, as a way to cope, I have stationed myself in my kitchen and focused on cooking. I have become a more adventurous cook, incorporating family recipes that I learned from Mom into our daily cuisine and borrowing from the culture around me. A silver lining perhaps?

It has been eight years since Mom was diagnosed with Alzheimer's. At the writing of this book, though she had declined in her abilities, Mom continued to function with a guarded independence, walking unassisted, dressing and showering herself (with increased and watchful support), and she was able to tell us how she felt. Today, sadly, Mom resides in a closed Alzheimer's care facility. Her daily life is drastically diminished and routine, and she struggles to rise from her chair. She remains outgoing and friendly most days, and still enjoys our visits. Music is a welcome break from an otherwise vacuous existence. Her most prized possession is a pair of headphones which play her favorite songs from times gone by.

People with Alzheimer's can survive with the disease for as many as twenty years, but the average is eight to ten years.[1] That may not leave us much time to savor our relationship. I know that what awaits us—the inevitable physical and mental decline that is Alzheimer's—will continue to generate a range of emotions and reactions, hurdles that I must overcome, to learn again and again to give of myself knowing I may not receive anything from Mom in return.

I am ready for that challenge. I invite you along to face it with me.

---

[1] "Alzheimer's Stages: How the Disease Progresses," Mayo Clinic website, November 24, 2015.

In the Beginning

they ask when she was diagnosed
as if that was the beginning
as if one day one noticeable event one small
symptom drew our attention
and we could pinpoint the first moment
of her memory loss
beginning middle end
a logical concept—
we only know middle
time sliding through time
no evident trigger
no first domino
signs piling up
until they erupt into diagnosis
we try to create
beginning out of chaos
but chaos
already was

Chapter 1

In the Beginning

After my mom, Naomi, was diagnosed with Alzheimer's in 2010 at the age of sixty-nine, my dad, Jack, only a few years older, started cooking for the first time in his life. Through the painful realization that we were losing our beloved mother and wife, we found humor in the situation—Daddy had actually entered the kitchen!

"I should write a cookbook," he joked the first time he'd made dinner for the two of them.

"That's a good idea," I replied. "We can document your cooking attempts. Did you burn anything?"

"No," he answered indignantly. Then, with a smile, "just the water."

❧

If there was a way to capture the essence of my mom, it was through her cooking. Though in later years she'd become, in her own words, "lazy" about cooking, my childhood was filled with bountiful family dinners, Friday night meals featuring golden chicken soup, and mouthwatering holiday feasts. The kitchen was Mom's domain. I remember photos of my parents taken in the early years of their marriage that amusingly defined their two distinct worlds: Jack, the scientist, in his lab; Naomi, pregnant in the kitchen.

They'd both grown up in the rough East End of London. My dad had been as skinny as a rake as a young man, with haunting, intelligent eyes and the temperament of an artist unwilling to compromise his beliefs. Mom's cooking soon fattened him up, and by the time I came along, Daddy had started to lose his undernourished appearance.

Mom was a beauty from day one. Photos show her as a smiling toddler—a round, pleasing face, two large dimples, and eyes that crinkled when she laughed. Sitting for her engagement photo, Mom looked like a shapely model: legs casually crossed, head tilted at an angle, her dark hair framing her face. She projected an overwhelming optimism as to what the future held.

೭ン೩ン೩

Fast forward fifty years. It took almost two years before the doctors were willing to finally diagnose what was entirely evident to our eyes. Mom was suffering from increasing short-term memory loss and an inability to keep up with conversations. She misplaced objects like keys and lists, credit cards and bills in the most unlikely of places, and shopped for the same items over and over again. At times, her memory was as sharp as or sharper than ours. Yet at other moments she would ask the same question within the same minute, or forget what she had ordered from a waiter before it arrived.

Outwardly, Mom somehow remained herself. Her essence—the bubbly, talkative, good-natured woman—was still there. She could dress herself, make jokes, and sing along to her favorite music. But she could no longer cook well-balanced or tasty meals. A huge part of her identity—the nurturing mother and wife who gave love through her cooking, the strong mother from my childhood—was now in jeopardy. Soon after she was diagnosed, Mom entered a more defined stage of Alzheimer's, what the Alzheimer's Association calls Moderate Severe Cognitive Decline. We knew that as an otherwise healthy seventy-year-old, Mom had many years of good health—and utter confusion—ahead of her.

Alzheimer's is one of the most common forms of dementia. A neurological brain dysfunction first described in 1906, it is characterized by an abnormal production of Amyloid beta in the brain's neurons. Amyloid beta begins to accumulate and binds to itself forming sticky aggregates called plaques that impair the normal functioning of our neurotransmitters. At the same time, a neural transporting protein called Tau undergoes anomalous chemical changes forming threads that clump together to create tangles. Both these processes halt the neurons' abilities to send and receive messages within the brain. What follows is an inability to access memories, and a gradual decline in cognitive and intellectual performance.[2] It also produces physical symptoms including loss of balance, difficulty walking, loss of smell, and vision impairment. Alzheimer's is progressive and irreversible and eventually leads to death. There is currently no cure.

---

[2] Genova, L, Lisa: "What You Can Do to Prevent Alzheimer's [video file]," TED Talks, ted.com, April 28, 2018

Alzheimer's intensifies the forgetfulness that occurs during the aging process. As we age, we sometimes forget words and names. Or we walk into a room and forget what we're looking for. Such "senior moments" may last a few moments before we retrieve the word or task that's eluded us. This is a normal part of aging. Alzheimer's sufferers are not so lucky. Alzheimer's patients may have trouble completing simple tasks, or misplace items in strange locations and be unable to find them later. They may stop communicating on a basic level. They'll sit quietly while a conversation is held around them. Familiar places become mazes, even within their own homes.

The kitchen is an especially forbidding room with its strange contraptions, appliances with indistinguishable buttons, or tomatoes that look like apples. The realization that they cannot manage a simple task can send an Alzheimer's patient into trembling bouts of fear and anger. Their emotions become amplified, and they may become confused, anxious, or suspicious, often toward those who are closest to them.

In Mom's case, the first thing to go was driving. By mutual consent, Daddy and Mom decided that the aggravation and anxiety Mom was feeling towards the car was not worth it. She called Daddy in tears from the parking lot under their building, unable to locate or unlock the alarm panel that was right next to her. Thankfully, my parents live in a city that is easy to navigate by foot. Grocery stores, clothing outlets, and a lively mall are all a short walk away. In the other direction, there's an outdoor pedestrian mall with restaurants, two community stages, and the sea twinkling invitingly beyond.

Next to go was the ability to consistently recognize ingredients needed in any given recipe. Mom took out two pieces of sole to defrost, then insisted it was chicken and refused to believe otherwise. She forgot how to cut vegetables for a salad. She burnt the toast almost every morning. She put pre-cooked chicken cutlets in the microwave then set the timer for *ten* minutes, making them completely inedible.

It was at this point that Daddy finally noticed the state of their kitchen. Early Alzheimer's patients often have a sense that they are forgetting to accomplish some task or other. For Mom, walking to the store to buy a couple of items she thought she needed became this task, one she felt she could accomplish with relative ease. But by the time she had reached the store, Mom would either have lost her list or couldn't remember what she had wanted to buy. She would buy, instead, those items that tickled her memory. Tuna cans, packages of chocolate cookies, bananas, canned olives, tomato sauce, toilet paper, and toothpaste were all stacked aplenty on her shelves. Once, she came home with an extra bag of fresh tomatoes thinking they were red peppers. Another time she bought a loaf of fresh bread, though the one she'd bought only the day before was still wrapped and sitting on the counter untouched.

When she forgot how to walk the few blocks home, she stopped going to the store by herself.

British by birth, my parents drink numerous cups of tea daily; yet Mom forgot how to make it. If she remembered how to boil the water, chances were she'd screw up making the tea. More than once she stuck a cookie into the cup as a substitute for a tea bag. Instead of taking tasks away from her, like making tea, Daddy and I tried to find solutions to her poor memory that would keep her feeling useful. For example, Mom was encouraged to wash the dishes, even though I often had to wash them again when she was done. When we made soup together, I would show Mom how to cut vegetables so that she could be part of the cooking process. Daddy hung whiteboards on each of the cupboards so that he could list their contents to help Mom find things she needed. He began to oversee the various tasks she was once able to accomplish herself. They prepared her medicines together, and Daddy helped her take them each morning and evening. They wrote the grocery list and kept it in a set place, adding to it as the days passed.

Meanwhile, my inbox was filling up with messages from Daddy about his growing cooking prowess. Daddy was learning to create delicious meals in under ten minutes. He was moving beyond omelets to other challenges. He made pasta with simple variations. He even tried chicken breasts with mushroom and white wine sauce!

I was also receiving emails from him about my mom's misadventures. "Today Naomi decided to make eggs in the microwave. Do you know what happens to an egg cooked in a microwave for more than two minutes? It literally explodes, and the resulting 'egg' resembles a hard plastic thing, more like a hockey puck than an actual egg. I've decided to call her 'the Egg Slayer.'"

Or: "Tonight I suggested we eat the leftover soup from last night. Before I had a chance to heat it up, Naomi added to it by dumping two jars of pasta sauce into the pot.

"It ceased being soup and became a thick sludge of tomato paste. She ate her share, but I opted to open a jar of gefilte fish instead."

For their fiftieth wedding anniversary in the summer of 2011, my parents took us all on a Mediterranean cruise. As getting lost on the ship would be frightfully easy for Mom, we promised to stick with her wherever she went. One evening, relaxing in the large lobby with the grandkids dancing round, she leaned over to Daddy and asked, "How many children did I give birth to?"

Such comments and actions caught us off guard. They pained and humored us, and gave us an inkling of what was to come. *How will we manage*, I wondered, *how will we take care of Mom?* As the child living in closest proximity to my parents, I felt the burden of caring for both of them acutely, for if Mom was not functioning, Daddy and I would have to pick up the slack.

The wealth of information online from the various Alzheimer's organizations only served to scare me. Was it safe to leave Mom alone? At what point would we have to make decisions without Mom's input? What would happen when she could no longer dress herself or use the bathroom? What if she became verbally or physically violent? What if she got lost? How much time did we have left? Were we strong enough to find the blessings in caring for an Alzheimer's patient?

Beyond the physical, Mom's emotional state was uppermost in our minds. What we knew in our hearts, what we'd realized all along, was that Mom's condition was only going to deteriorate. We braced ourselves for the stages to come and watched as she vacillated between anger and fear.

❧❧❧

"You're right, we *should* write a cookbook," I said to Daddy in one of our many conversations. I was looking for a way to overcome the growing despondency I felt towards my mom's condition. It seemed a logical extension of the hours I'd devoted to helping him learn to cook. I envisioned a humorous account of my dad's growth in the kitchen and how his experience was probably being played out in thousands of kitchens across the globe—men who had matured in an age when male and female roles were so well defined, the best they could do was make scrambled eggs or put together a slap-dash sandwich. And now, here he was, stepping into his wife's shoes because she could no longer cook for him. The idea of creating a cookbook together based on Daddy's culinary experiences began to take shape. We opted to title it, *The Man's Emergency Cookbook.*

We did start a project together, but at some point, I realized that what I needed to say had become much broader than the confining theme we had set for ourselves. With a small shudder at separating our work, I decided to continue the project on my own.

With Daddy's blessing, I worked to transcend the emotional burden of my mom's Alzheimer's through my creativity. My father's fanciful comment had become a medium for me.

૭౨౭౨

It would be impossible to describe my early years without mentioning the kitchen in which I grew up. Everything happened in our kitchen. With its orange-flowered walls, yellow curtains, and gleaming brown fridge, the kitchen was a warm place to gather. We each had our assigned seats around the butcher block table that was nestled in the breakfast nook: Mom and Daddy along one edge, my brother Simon and I each at one of the ends. I would sit for hours in those heavy oak chairs, back against the wall, feet resting on the stretcher bar under the seat, reading all manner of books. The radio was always on tuned to rock or classical depending on who got to it first. Here was the source of my informal education about music and the world. I remember listening to Rossini's "William Tell Overture" with its grand, romping finale; and, when I finally understood them, being scandalized by lyrics to popular songs such as Dylan's

"Lay, Lady, Lay." On Sunday mornings, we'd hear "Awake, Alive, and Jewish," a staple of the local community broadcasts.

And Mom was there, a fixture by the counter: cutting, chopping, stirring. The kitchen was a good place to be.

If we begin at the very beginning, I would plumb one of my earliest memories to describe the dish Mom made whenever we children were sick. She'd mash a banana in a small bowl, add one-fourth cup of milk and two teaspoons of sugar. The riper the banana, the better the taste. Something about the lumpy consistency or the mushy, sweetened milk always made me feel better.

I remember being put to bed in the middle of the day at age five or six, with several heavy blankets to reduce my fever by sweating it out. When I woke hours later, the fever gone, Mom fed me mashed bananas.

Mom didn't work outside of the house until my brother Simon and I were in our last years of grade school. Though I didn't understand or even realize it at the time, she battled a sense of inadequacy because she didn't have a university degree. She was married to a PhD in chemistry from Cambridge University, but she herself had been forced to give up a college career. You could blame it on her family's lack of money, or on the fact that when she was young, most women did not pursue degrees. Or you could lay the blame squarely at the feet of my grandmother, who, with her extreme old-world views on modesty and dating, ripped up Mom's letter of admission to study languages at Birmingham University, without telling her she'd been accepted, and sent her to typing school instead.

My grandmother's cooking fame was largely epitomized by the statement: "I treat my husband like a god—I give him burnt offerings." Fortunately, Mom ultimately learned many things on her own, including how to cook.

The most fundamental essence of Mom, however, was captured in her chicken soup. This soup was always Mom's expression of love for our family. She cooked this dish with only fresh herbs and vegetables cut into big chunks. We delighted in the clear, golden broth, the tender strands of chicken, soft celery and aromatic dill. It was the highlight of every Friday night meal when I was growing up. Later, when my husband Jeff and I visited with our kids, the kids always requested seconds, and sometimes even thirds of her fragrant liquid. For this dish, the secret to success is the fresh dill.

Naomi's Golden Chicken Soup

Don't even think about using dried herbs for this soup. Do think about adding extra chicken parts to make sure there's enough to satisfy you when your guests request their second and third bowls.

1 thigh, 1 breast, 2 legs of chicken
1½ onions, quartered
2 carrots, sliced
1 potato, chopped
2 small turnips, chopped
2 celery stalks, chopped
3-4 sprigs fresh parsley
3-4 sprigs fresh dill
6 cups water (may use more)
Salt and pepper to taste

Directions:
Chop vegetables into large chunks. Set aside. In a large pot, boil chicken in water. When chicken is cooked, remove and let cool. Skim the top of the water to remove any fat. Add vegetables, salt, and pepper. Add three to four whole sprigs of parsley and dill. Debone chicken and return to the pot without the bones. Bring to a boil then simmer for several hours.

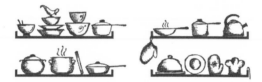

Winter Rain

We wait for the rain
that beats the Land like a tight drum,
tense with expectation
for the tenacious downpour.
I watch from my window as the streaks
of sand that have gathered all summer
are slowly vanquished.
Now it pours in wide sheets
as clear as if the rain were a portal
that I could step through.
The air is crisp with a brisk chill
and bright hail begins to crack
against the roof
and the solar panels
that are made of thick glass.
I want to make my palms into a scooped bowl,
gather the rain in my hands.
I want to share it with my mom
who sits by a window,
the rivulets sluicing through her fogged brain,
its restorative powers
no match for Alzheimer's.
Now the water overwhelms the parched Land
surging in a powerful wave
through dry wadis to the Dead Sea.
Everything in its path—trees, boulders, cars,
people—vanish
in the churning mud.

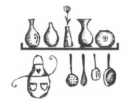
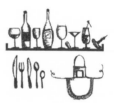

Chapter 2

My Mother, My Teacher

By the time she gave me all her cookbooks, Mom had almost entirely stopped cooking. She still made sandwiches for lunch, and endless cups of tea, but her more extensive culinary skills had dwindled to zero. We didn't know exactly what "stage" of Alzheimer's she had entered, but we recognized it as another in a series of declines.

With Daddy cooking on a daily basis, we joked that he had found his true passion. After years of being a chemist, he'd brought his scientific expertise into the kitchen. And Mom deserved to sit back and let him do the work after all her years of service.

As a reaction to Mom's diagnosis, I made a commitment to visit my parents on a weekly basis. The idea was to provide as much support as I could as their lives slowly changed. Not only did I want to comfort Mom through this emotional turmoil, but I wanted to counter Daddy's initial desire to ignore or pull Mom back—often painfully and in anger—from her altering reality. I arranged my schedule so that I could visit my parents in their home in Netanya—a coastal city in Israel—every Tuesday. My challenge was to keep Mom occupied so that Daddy could have a break.

It was a long haul. I'd take the seven a.m. train from Beer Sheva to Tel Aviv, grab a shared taxi at the train station, and arrive in Netanya by nine-thirty a.m. My parents would meet me at the central bus station, and then Mom and I would make our way to my Grandmother Millie's nursing home. When she turned ninety-seven, Booba, as we called her, didn't remember that it was her birthday. Mom, bless her, knowing our birthdays were back-to-back, asked in all seriousness if I was turning eighteen. (No need to remind her—or myself—that I was almost fifty!) As I watched Millie's 24/7 Philippine caregiver washing, dressing, and diapering my grandmother, I kept thinking that soon we'd need to provide this service for Mom, too.

In some ways, she was already lost to me. The mother who had comforted me, taken an interest in my activities, and shaped my knowledge of motherhood, now seemed younger and less capable than I was.

Even something innocuous like saying the "Grace after Meals," a blessing that religious Jews recite after they eat a meal with bread, became problematic. As I sat at Mom's table, I recited: "God of compassion, bless my father and my mother, my teachers, hosts of this household." At first, I felt sad saying those words. Was Mom still my teacher? How could she be? She had taught me many things when I was growing up, some quite practical (how to check eggs in a carton before you buy them), others intangible (that children thrive when you love them unconditionally). But now?

Still, I looked forward to Tuesdays. I saved my errands so that Mom and I would have some direction to our wanderings. We had fun together! We roamed the bustling streets of Netanya window shopping and telling jokes, laughing at all manner of things around us. We stopped for coffee and sipped our drinks in view of the azure Mediterranean. I tried hard to keep our outings stress free. If it meant bending the truth to fit Mom's reality, that's what I did. Sometimes, she informed me she was only forty-six, making me the older of us two. Or she'd say, puzzled, "Daddy went to work and hasn't called all day." I could never tell if she were referring to my dad, who's been retired for years, or her dad, who, sadly, passed away nineteen years ago. Often, she'd ask where "Jack" was, thinking he was a different person from "Daddy." If I tried explaining that "Daddy" and her husband Jack were the same person, she would utterly reject it. It was easier to lie. "Oh, I spoke to him today. He's fine. He'll be home soon."

"But what has he been doing?" she'd ask.

"You can ask him when you see him," I'd suggest, thereby setting up an open-ended conversation we replayed many times.

Sometimes she'd admit to being frightened by her memory loss. Other times she wanted to be held. The first time she came into my arms, I felt awkward. She hugged me tight and cried against my chest. I gave her comfort, of course, but I realized my role of child was shifting. What I wanted—to remain her child—could not last.

As a memory exercise, I tried to get her to remember how to prepare some of my favorite dishes that she had made while we were growing up. Clarity would often elude her, though on some days, she'd give me exact measurements and describe the cooking process without hesitation.

There was one recipe I never did succeed in discovering. I remember a luscious trout dish with roasted al-

17

monds, grapes and a creamy cheese stuffing. It was absent from all of Mom's cookbooks, and she never remembered the dish when I prodded her about it.

I do believe that Mom is still teaching me new things. I am learning to accept her reality, to explore ways of stimulating her and keeping her active. I am learning that time can shift as past memories become the present; and that laughter is a precious commodity. I am learning the art of patience. And I am learning to let go of the frustration I feel in losing myself when I am with her.

છ∕જ∕જ

My earliest memories are tied to my early childhood years in Israel, and it is no wonder that at a certain age I was sure I'd live there one day. Experiencing discomfort in my American homeland may also have contributed to that decision.

Like many Jewish families, ours is a mixture of cultures and traditions. Three of my grandparents were born in England while the fourth arrived there as a young boy. *Their* families had come from Poland, the Ukraine, and Holland, all escaping the devastation that befell those Jews who stayed behind. My parents were born in England, and likewise my brother Simon and I; while we were still toddlers, we moved to the US for career and economic considerations, first to New Jersey and then to Maryland.

For all intents and purposes, I was a typical American kid. We lived in the suburbs and attended the local schools. It's true that I hated peanut butter, and my parents had a strange accent, but I learned to appreciate the holidays and freedoms of my adopted country. And yet I *was* different. By the fact of my foreign parents and by my Jewish birth, I was other. I attended Hebrew school, most days quite reluctantly. I had uncontrollable wavy hair, braces, and awkwardness in social circles. I saw myself as the antithesis of the all-American kid. In second grade, my gracious teacher awarded me the "Question Award" for the many questions I pondered and asked, setting me on a path to claim an identity I did not see reflected around me.

The American culture was new to all of us. I remember the first time I helped carve a pumpkin with my neighbor Carla Flowers, thrusting my arms into the dark orange insides to scoop out handfuls of slimy white seeds. Drinking Coke, that most American of all drinks, was a torture: the bubbles invariably rose up my nose and I would start coughing and spluttering. I learned to sip it slowly to avoid embarrassment.

From the moment they arrived, my parents blossomed in the America in which we found ourselves. Entrenched within the Jewish community of Greater Washington, they made friends, and became active in the Soviet Jewry movement, an international human rights campaign that advocated for the right of Russian Jews to emigrate. Mom, in particular, found confidence to attend community college and take on increasingly responsible positions, rising before her retirement to Executive Director of our local synagogue. Daddy pursued his science with the same intensity that he did everything else: a mindfulness that propelled him to head several institutes within the National Cancer Institute at NIH, the National Science Foundation, and Georgetown University.

They obviously had an easier time than I at acculturating. I remember a summer day at Camp Breezy Hollow on the grounds of the National Institutes of Health, which was run for the kids of employees, where the counselors I had befriended chose me to play Frankenstein's bride in a skit. They teased my already curly hair into a horrible mess, painted my face in shades of green and white, and dressed me in a long robe. It was fun to be the center of attention; I was a star. When I saw myself in the mirror, I burst into tears. They had unintentionally made me as other and as separate as I already felt. I had been betrayed by their joyful enthusiasm. I couldn't explain to Mom what it was that so upset me. She took me back to camp the next day—they were both working full time jobs—but my initial enthusiasm at being there waned. To this day I cringe at how I saw myself in their eyes.

In 1976, we spent a year in Israel. I was twelve. We slept beneath musky orange blossoms and hiked the coarse, needy country. From the edges to the center of identity, my worldview was formed by the daring rescue at Entebbe, Israel's basketball victory in Europe, the strains of *Hatikva,*[3] and a novel called *Smith's Gazelle.*[4] I spent long days reading anything I could get my hands on. I plowed through James Michener's *The Source,*[5] and as much writing by Herman Wouk and Leon Uris as I could find. I returned to the US with confidence to know who I wanted to be and to make writing a priority. And I pledged to return to Israel.

It was a difficult reentry for me when we moved back to our house in Maryland. I had missed seventh grade, that transition year to junior high, boys, and the unspoken dress and conduct code. Mom guided me as best she could, but she couldn't protect me from the cruelty of former friends who had moved on without me.

By the time I graduated high school, I had figured out how to navigate the problematic social scene on my own, mostly by arranging my life outside of those hall-

---

[3] Israel's national anthem.
[4] Davidson, Lionel, *Smith's Gazelle,* UK, Jonathan Cape, 1971.
[5] Michener, James, *The Source,* Random House, US, 1965.

ways. And I had acquitted myself by becoming editor of the high school newspaper. Finding the right college, though, was another hurdle made difficult by our immigrant status.

I returned to Israel in 1982 as part of a post-high school year abroad with a deferment to Oberlin College tucked safely in my pocket. It was a year of dramatic emotional experiences that taught me that Israel was a country to which I belonged, though not necessarily on a kibbutz like the one on which my group had been living. Arriving in Oberlin, I sought out other students who were wearing Israeli sandals, recognizing in them a link to my future.

When I finally moved to Israel in 1991, my brother Simon was already settled in California. "My daughter moved to one promised land, and my son to the other," Daddy told friends. In the winter of 1993, Mom slipped on the ice on her front porch, broke her wrist and declared, "Enough! No more winters in Maryland!" A year later, they, too, arrived in Israel, just in time for the birth of their first grandchild.

My husband Jeff and I celebrated our first wedding anniversary in Beer Sheva. It was shortly after the first Gulf War, and Rosh Hashana fell early that year. We had the feeling that the whole country was celebrating with us as we marked the exciting embodiment of our Zionist dreams one year into a loving, stable relationship. To this day, I picture us as young adventurers walking hand-in-hand down the quiet streets as holiday candles cast their glow through open windows.

Three children, two cats, a pet snake, and twenty-eight years later, we are still going strong. I have no doubt at all that my ability to visit my parents on a weekly basis rests on Jeff's support and encouragement to give them all I can as they age. He helps around the house, makes chicken soup, tells (mostly) funny jokes, keeps his moustache trim, volunteers at our synagogue, learns and teaches Torah several nights a week, washes dishes, folds laundry, gives of himself to our children, and generally brings optimism to our household.

❧❧❧

Israel is a nation of immigrants. The cultural cues we misunderstand are repeated *ad nauseam* by the constant wave of immigrants arriving here. My children are in good company in that respect, as many of their friends are also the offspring of immigrants. In a country the size of Delaware, it is easier to make connections and navigate the foreign shores.

I know I am blessed to have my parents living relatively close to me in Israel. As my knowledge of Hebrew increases, I find myself becoming their bridge to understanding the countless medical forms and letters that they are bombarded with. One of the hard parts about visiting them once a week is that my children have needs, too. I'm a typical member of the sandwich generation, those sandwiched between aging parents who need care and/or help, and their own children. I know my children will forgive me for the days I am absent caring for my parents. As they lead their own busy lives, they need my mothering less and less. I want them to know that I am always here for them, but right now, my parents are my priority. Mom's laughter—our mutual joy at being together—won't go on indefinitely. That's why I visit every week.

Israel has greatly influenced our cuisine: we make a salad of cucumber and tomatoes cut into tiny pieces, we add pomegranate seeds to food, we cook with chickpeas, and humus is a staple on our table. The recipes that follow are a selection of those that reflect our changing taste buds.

Meat and Humus

Our dear friend Ken introduced us to this dish. Its combination of flavors is very Mediterranean.

1 lb / ½ kilo ground beef
1 onion, chopped
2 cloves garlic, crushed
2 Tbsp pine nuts
1 tsp coriander
1 tsp cumin
1½ cups humus (see adjacent recipe)

Directions:
Sauté onion and garlic. When onion becomes translucent, add meat. Brown meat and add spices and pine nuts. Simmer for another twenty minutes. Spoon humus into a serving dish. Hollow out a concave area in the middle, and pile meat on top. Serve hot with fresh pita bread.

Humus

Humus is one of those dishes that take on the personality of the maker. Dress it up with olive oil and paprika, zatar and sesame seeds, fried mushrooms and onions, or tehina. Or be totally Israeli and scoop it up with a pita fresh from the oven.

1 19-oz / 550-gr can pre-cooked chickpeas, drained
½ cup liquid from chickpea can
3 Tbsp raw tehina
1 tsp sesame oil
2 Tbsp lemon juice
2-3 cloves garlic
1 tsp cumin
Salt and pepper to taste

For garnish:
Paprika
¼ cup pine nuts

Directions:
Combine all ingredients in a food processor and blend until creamy. If mixture isn't blending, add a little more liquid. Place humus in a shallow bowl and, using a spoon, create an indentation in the middle of the bowl. Drizzle olive oil and paprika into the indentation. Add pine nuts for effect.

Moroccan Nile Perch

We love the subtle yet spicy taste of this fish. Once, my oldest son won a bet by eating one of the hot peppers. The pepper was green—but he turned red!

2 lbs / 1 kilo Nile perch cut into large 2" chunks,
or tilapia, amnon (St. Peter's), or salmon, 4-5 fillets
1½ red peppers, sliced
1 onion, sliced
2 small potatoes, thinly sliced
up to 4 small hot chili peppers sliced or whole
1 head garlic, peeled and whole
1 cup pre-cooked chick peas
2 cups water or enough to cover vegetables
2 Tbsp olive oil
2 Tbsp Moroccan paprika
Salt and pepper to taste
1 cup fresh cilantro, chopped
juice of one lemon

Directions:
Place fish in bowl with lemon juice and a sprinkling of salt and paprika. Let soak. In a large pan, sauté onions, garlic, potatoes, peppers and chick peas in oil with spices. After 10 minutes on a medium flame, add water and bring to a boil. Reduce heat and simmer uncovered for an additional 10 minutes or until potatoes begin to soften. Make room in pan for fish (without lemon liquid) under the vegetables and cook covered on a low flame for 20 minutes or until fish is cooked through. Remove from flame and stir in cilantro. Let cool slightly.

A note about hot peppers. Depending on how hot you like your dish, you can either slice the hot peppers and cook with the other vegetables or slit the peppers down the center and leave them whole for the duration of the cooking. How to decide. I always opt for the less hot dish but my Israeli children seem to have been born with a desire for spicy food. The best option is to taste one of the peppers before cooking to assess its fieriness.

A note about Moroccan paprika. Moroccan paprika is a traditional blend of freshly ground paprika, olive oil, sea salt and sometimes garlic. If you don't find it in your grocery store, use 1 Tbsp sweet paprika and 1 Tbsp hot paprika. And don't be shy about adding more if you so desire. When I made this dish with my daughter, she probably added an additional tablespoon!

Serve this dish on a bed of couscous. Couscous is a traditional dish of semolina (granules of durum wheat) that is cooked by steaming. We make it the easy way by buying it pre-cooked in the freezer section of our grocery store. If that's not available, buy it in packages that are located next to the rice in many supermarkets; add water and spices according to directions, and it's ready within five minutes.

Roasted Eggplant and Tehina

Eggplant is frequently served in Israel, and in many ways: fried, smoked, mashed, grilled, roasted and baked. It took me a while to warm to this vegetable, but now that I know the secret to roasting eggplants, I enjoy making this dish. Unprocessed tehina is sold as a paste in plastic containers. It makes a flavorful dip or spread.

1 large eggplant
Salt
¼ cup fresh parsley, chopped
1 tsp date honey
1 tsp rosemary

Tehina:
½ cup unprocessed tehina
½ cup water
¼ cup olive oil
2 cloves garlic, crushed
3 Tbsp lemon juice
Salt and pepper to taste

Directions:
Cut eggplant in half lengthwise and score the fleshy inside in a cross hatch. Cut as deeply as you can, then sprinkle with salt, letting sit for half an hour. Dry eggplant to remove moisture. Brush with olive oil and sprinkle with rosemary. Place cut side down on a baking sheet. Bake at 420 degrees F / 210 degrees C for twenty minutes until eggplant is completely soft, even slightly browned. Remove from oven and let cool. Meanwhile mix tehina in a small bowl. When eggplants are cool, turn cut side up on a serving dish, drizzle with tehina, date honey, and fresh parsley.

Roasted Eggplant and Pepper Salad

Here's another of our favorite eggplant dishes. For a truly Israeli experience, substitute amba for the mustard. Amba is a tangy mango chutney that takes its name from the Sanskrit word for mango.

1 large eggplant, sliced
1½ red peppers, halved
1 large tomato, chopped
¼ onion, finely diced
¼ cup fresh parsley, chopped

Dressing:
2-3 cloves garlic, crushed
2 Tbsp olive oil
2 Tbsp lemon juice
1 Tbsp mustard
1 Tbsp vinegar
¼ tsp hot pepper flakes
Salt and pepper to taste

Directions:
Cut eggplant in ½ inch (1 cm) slices and sprinkle with salt, letting sit for at least half an hour. Dry each slice with a towel to remove moisture. Brush eggplant slices and pepper halves with olive oil and place on a large baking tray, peppers cut side down. Bake at 420 degrees F / 210 degrees C for twenty minutes or until pepper skins start to blacken and eggplant can be easily pierced with a knife. Let cool. Peel skins from peppers. Chop tomato, peppers, and eggplant and combine with diced onion and garlic. Add parsley. In a small container, whisk dressing ingredients. Combine with vegetables. Serve cold.

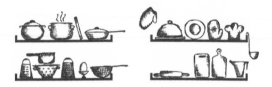

It's Getting Worse

She thinks her apartment is not her real home.
By her calculation, I'm older than she is.
She mistakes Daddy for *her* father.
She wears the same shirt
three days in a row. I help her dress
when she puts her underwear on backward.
She tells me I am her best sister—
I don't correct her. That dream
where she pulls me out of bed
by my hair and doesn't know me.
When I wake in a sweat,
she is still asleep in the next room.

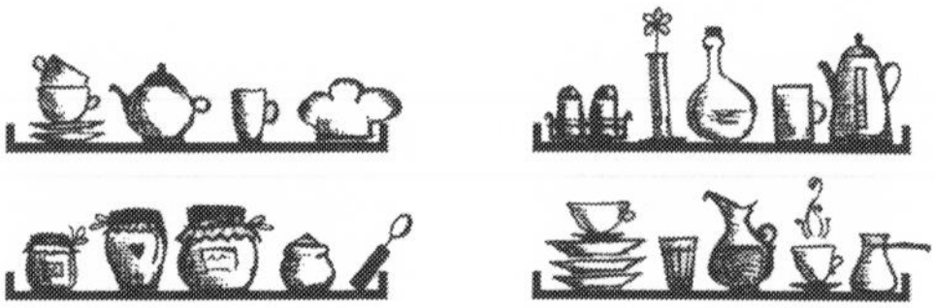

Chapter 3

Shadowing

When my three kids, Rafi, Liora, and Hillel, were little, we went on many family vacations overseas. Most were to the US, where the bulk of our relatives still resided. It was important for us to keep our family close, despite the geographic distance that divided us. With my brother Simon in California, Europe became an alternative destination for family gatherings where we might meet up and explore new vistas. We visited Florence and Rome in 2009, then went on a Mediterranean cruise in 2011. But it was our trip to London in the summer of 2014 that nearly brought the house down.

We could see it so clearly. Mom was exhibiting "shadowing" behavior. Four years after her diagnosis, Simon, his wife Sharon, and their daughter Shoshana came from the US and met us in London for a family heritage tour of our birth city. Though we were uprooting Mom from her everyday routines, we thought London would evoke positive early childhood memories for her. It soon became clear that she was out of her element.

Everywhere Daddy went, Mom was sure to go. If he rode the London underground, Mom stood right next to him. If he took a boat ride down the Thames, Mom sat so she could see him. If he went up to his room in our rented house, she would follow. And if she couldn't see him, she became agitated. This is the essence of "shadowing:" the caregiver becomes the touchstone—like a parent for a young child—to an Alzheimer's patient who can no longer navigate the world on her own. She tries to keep her caregiver in her sight at all times. Unfortunately for the caregiver, this often produces a feeling of resentment at losing all personal space.

Surprisingly, Mom seemed to remember each grandchild, though she fumbled on their ages. The kids had overcome their fears about dealing with her dementia when they realized she still had her same broad smile and happy laugh. But she couldn't remember where we were, what day it was, what season it was, or who any of our extended family members were.

One conversation was particularly jarring. Mom's sister Barbara and her son Mark, who both live in London, had come to visit and we were sitting together talking. I mentioned that the last time Mark had been to Israel was when our grandfather had died.

"*Zaida is dead?*" Mom exclaimed.

The obvious distress in her voice made us all turn to her as one, incredulity written all over our faces. Her sadness at her father's death—an event that had taken place nineteen years previously—was shocking, even to us Alzheimer-scarred veterans. Our conversation stopped in its tracks. We cautiously started a different conversation, and by mutual agreement, my Zaida's death became a taboo subject in her presence. I didn't want Mom to experience that loss again.

On the first part of our trip, we went on some amazing outings: visiting St. Catherine's College in Cambridge where Daddy had received his PhD, with a punt ride along the river Cam; touring the Tower of London with a funny, irreverent Beefeater; and shaking the hand of Henry VIII in Hampton Court. And, of course, we shopped in Camden Market.

One of the best days included a performance of Shakespeare's *Macbeth* at the Globe, the replica of the original Elizabethan theatre, where the actors perform in the open air. My youngest was bored to tears but the rest of us found the play engaging. Mom was especially engrossed. In fact, she remembered much of the play line-by-line from having learned it in grammar school. She spoke the actors' lines often before they spoke them on stage! The audience sitting around us was understandably annoyed by her antics, but I was secretly excited by her active memory.

Then it all crumbled. Back at the house where we were staying, Daddy appeared at my door and said he couldn't take it anymore. He and Mom had had a fight. After he had suggested she wear different clothes that morning instead of the ones she'd worn the day before, she became abusive, shouting at him to stop telling her what to do. She'd exhibited anger in the past, but never with such vehemence. She hit him, cursed like a sailor, and yelled that he might as well put her away in a home. The childish dependency that had compelled her to shadow him everywhere had now transformed into an equally childish rage. Daddy pushed her into my arms, then stormed into his room and locked the door.

It took a long time to comfort Mom. In her heightened emotional state, she was nervous that Daddy would leave her because she'd yelled at him. Contrite, she wanted to apologize immediately. But I told her that Daddy needed time alone. We took a long walk, sat on a park bench, and she fell asleep in my arms, as vulnerable as a baby. I marveled at my ability to keep her safe, but I was heartbroken to realize I'd lost my mom again.

They worked through the anger but it was agreed that I had to take on more of the immediate burden of caring for Mom. As each day drew to a close, I'd stop by their room to help her pick out clothes for the next day. We'd chat about where we were and our plans for the day ahead. Most of London was as foreign to Mom as it was to the rest of us, but suddenly, as we drove through Stamford Hill, Mom's long-term memory kicked in. She recognized her childhood neighborhood with surprising clarity, calling out the names of the roads as we drove by and chatting about her girlhood.

The difficulties of trying to enjoy ourselves on vacation in a new environment while caring for Mom's needs was trying on all of us; we decided that this was the last time Mom would be traveling outside of Israel.

℘℘℘

Throughout Mom's Alzheimer's, I have made it a priority to include her as much as possible in the cycle of our family celebrations—Passover Seders, Rosh Hashanah meals, birthdays and once-in-a-lifetime events like my son's wedding in 2014. Mom thought of my oldest as a little kid rather than a young man on the cusp of his marriage. Plus, traveling anywhere, even within Israel, unsettled Mom's sense of familiarity and well-being.

In the weeks leading up to Rafi's wedding, it was fun to tell Mom each time we met that Rafi was about to get married. I'd show her the invitation and we'd count the days. She'd ask me about his bride, and I'd tell her how Rafi and Hadas had met through their youth group, and that they'd been going out since high school. "Have I met Hadas?" she'd ask, though the answer was obvious.

The morning after the wedding, it was already lost. Getting dressed in our finest clothes, putting on make-up, walking into the beautifully decorated hall. The emotional meeting of bride and groom after a week's separation, the way Rafi cried with love and anticipation as he performed the *bedeken*, the veiling ceremony, and watched Hadas walk towards him under the *chuppah*, the wedding canopy. The *freilich* joyous dancing, the hugs and kisses from friends and family. All of it gone, as if none of it had happened.

If I'd learned anything about Alzheimer's, it was that though Mom's past might be lost, and her future was, well, non-existent, her present was immediate. Every moment that she spent at the wedding was fully experienced. One of the absolute highlights in an evening of amazing experiences was when we presented Mom with a birthday cake for her seventy-third birthday. The band came over and played "Happy Birthday" then seamlessly switched to swing music. Daddy grabbed Mom's hands and that was it, they were dancing as they loved to do, twisting and twirling together in fluid motion. The whole hall clapped and watched, and nothing else existed at that moment.

That was one of the lessons I have been trying to learn from her: live the now fully.

How did I feel? Exuberant! My son's wedding was filled with blessings. And sad. I was forced to acknowledge that even in the midst of the life-affirming wedding, I inhabited a space between my son and mother. I had launched Rafi into a new stage in his life, pushing him to spread his wings and find himself. Meanwhile,

Mom seemed to be growing more and more childlike. So many people said hello to her at the wedding. She kept asking me who they were, how I knew them, what they were doing there. The trick was to stay patient and keep smiling. As sad as I was inside, being with Mom did not have to be sad. Mom was a happy Alzheimer's individual. For the most part, we could enjoy ourselves together, regardless of the circumstances.

I had several conversations that weekend that stayed with me for a long while. One was with my cousin Mark who spoke about the death of his father, my beloved Uncle Malcolm: "While you're going through it, you don't think about what you're doing. You just do it. And you don't think of yourself with pity. Afterward, you look at your hands and you ask yourself, 'Did I really bathe and feed my father? Did I really take care of him in such an intimate way?'"

Another with my sister-in-law Sharon who has a degree in gerontology: "There are so many ways you can approach Alzheimer's. Your mom is full of life. She is a pleasure to be with, and that's what you have to focus on."

One of the hardest conversations was with my brother: "I don't know when I'm coming back. At this rate, Mom might not recognize or remember me. Her sentences and thoughts are becoming so disconnected."

Simon lives in California, I live in Israel. There is a lot of geographical distance between us. "I'm sorry I'm not here to help you more," he said.

He does help, though. He calls daily to speak with Mom, and he visits as often as he can. He even made her a pictorial family tree for her to identify her kids and grandkids. I told him it wasn't worth being sorry, that regrets are the past, and the past was over. But I was sorry. I was sorry he'd miss the joy of being with Mom while she was still so present. Nothing can replace that as she slips into forgetfulness.

Baking Challah

In preparation for the family Shabbat after the wedding, I took the time to bake challah, traditional bread eaten on Shabbat and other Jewish holidays. My signature challah is a combination of white dough and whole wheat dough arranged in a circular baking pan with sesame seeds sprinkled on top. I also like to braid challah with four-strands. When you make challah every week, you start to sense how the dough will turn out. If you are trying challah for the first time, there are a few tricks you can employ to make sure it turns out well.

1. Adding a little oil to your hands allows you to knead the dough without it sticking.

2. If it is too sticky, add more flour.

3. Whole wheat flour needs more water than white flour to become dough. Don't be shy about adding more than the recipe calls for, but add it in small amounts.

4. Let dough rise in a warm place like the top of the refrigerator.

5. If the dough hasn't risen much after two hours, kneed it, shape it, and when you're ready to bake it, bake at a low temp for about ten minutes before you turn up the oven to 350 degrees F / 180 degrees C.

For the two-toned white and brown challah effect, you need to make this recipe twice, once with white flour and once with whole wheat flour. Most weeks, I make a batch of white challah to satisfy my family's preference.

Challah

2.2 lbs / 1 kilo white and/or whole wheat flour
1 cup sugar (can use brown sugar)
1 Tbsp yeast
1 Tbsp salt
1 egg for the dough
1 egg for brushing on top
1½ to 2 cups warm water
½ cup vegetable oil
Sesame seeds

Directions:
In a large bowl, proof yeast by adding ½ cup of sugar and one cup water to yeast. Let sit for about twenty minutes. Add flour, remaining sugar, salt, and egg to yeast mixture. Add in water and oil. Using your hands, mix until a small ball of dough forms. (Don't be afraid to add a little more water and/or oil to create the dough, preferably a handful at a time.) Lift dough out of bowl and knead on a floured surface until dough becomes uniform. Return dough to bowl and coat with a thin layer of oil. (This is the point at which you take "challah.") Cover bowl and let rise in a warm location for two hours. Dough will expand in size. Punch down and knead dough until all air bubbles are gone. Divide and shape dough into braided or rounded challahs. Place on baking sheet (covered with baking paper) and let rise at least another hour in a warm location. Just before baking, brush top of challah with beaten egg and sprinkle with sesame seeds. Makes four *challot*. Bake at 350 degrees F / 180 degrees C for twenty minutes or until bread becomes golden brown.

Taking Challah

This is one of the 613 *mitzvot*, commandments, that observant Jews follow. When we first moved to Israel, our neighbors were the local rabbi and his wife. They were the sweetest, kindest of people, and it is from Rabbi Aharon and Leah Rabenstein that I learned when to take challah with a blessing, and when to take it without a blessing. May their memories, too, be for a blessing.

There are differing halachic opinions as to what amount of flour you use that constitutes enough for taking challah with and without a bracha. For more information on this mitzvah, visit "A Taste of Challah," a website created by Tamar Ansch, a friend and author of *A Taste of Challah.*[6]

---

[6] Ansch, Tamar, *A Taste of Challah,* Feldheim Books, 2007

Confession

She swore like a sailor,
called herself a cunt,

hit her own legs and arms,
cried, said she didn't mean it,

wanted to apologize immediately,
all those words

she'd branded my father,
worried he would leave her,

confessed she did forget sometimes.
I held her, smoothed her hair,

wiped her tears with my hand.
She sat with me on the bench as if

I were her mother, head resting
in the crook of my arm, her body

slowly relaxing
like an infant heavy with sleep.

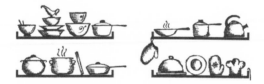

Chapter 4

Hiring a Caregiver

The phone calls came at odd hours, often while I was at work or eating dinner.

"Hi, darling," she'd say, "have you seen Daddy today? I haven't heard from him and I'm just so worried."

Sometimes Mom was alone while Daddy ran errands or attended meetings. Most of the time he was in the next room but Mom didn't identify him as her husband. As I was still visiting once a week, Daddy tried to arrange as many of his weekly meetings as he could on Tuesdays so I could be with Mom instead of her being alone. The remaining hours of each day Mom and Daddy were together. They attended lectures and concerts, visited with friends, or spent time in their apartment. But Mom's world was shrinking. Her ability to concentrate on books was quickly waning, and she couldn't keep TV characters straight in any given show. And now she was exhibiting anxiety over being alone.

Once, when I was about fifteen, we'd watched a particularly exciting cop movie. When it was over, Mom was confused. She couldn't figure out which of the actors were the FBI agents and which ones were the criminals. That became a running family joke. "Wait," we'd say after every movie, "which ones were the good guys?" We chalked it up to being an amusing quirk in Mom's personality that she could never keep the plot straight. We never dreamed it might eventually become something more pernicious.

As Mom's anxiety level rose at being left alone, Daddy and I decided it was time to hire a caregiver. I'd be there once a week, but other mornings had to be "covered" by someone so that Daddy had some time to himself. In theory, it sounded like a good plan. In practice, Mom was having none of it. Mom didn't want a caregiver. She didn't want someone taking away her independence or telling her what to do, and she certainly didn't want a stranger in her house. She could take care of herself.

Or could she? Well, yes, she could, but only to a certain extent, and even that was decreasing almost daily. Her perception of reality was changing. We started asking ourselves if Mom was competent enough to be part of the decision-making or whether it was time for us to make decisions for her. In my mind, the phone calls I kept receiving were gigantic sign-posts telling me that she could no longer decide for herself. Mom could still find and dial my number, but the conversations we held were riddled with inconsistencies. When Daddy asked their family physician for his opinion, he received the same advice—it's time to make decisions without her input. With regret, we bit the bullet and left her out of the loop.

It took several tries until we found the right person. The first woman we interviewed was too assertive. She decided they'd walk each morning whether Mom wanted to or not. Her tone was bossy, and Mom kept saying she didn't like her. The second regaled Mom with sad tales about her difficult life. Just what we needed. The third woman we tried was a keeper. We were delighted that Rachel had walked into our lives.

Rachel's job was to be Mom's companion. She was not there to assist with Mom's dressing or grooming or constant tea-making, but rather to be a friend. She delighted Mom with her ability to spin yarns and reference old movies. She was gentle and full of laughter. When Mom's anger flared over some perceived injustice, Rachel knew how to calm her. When Mom stormed away from her, Rachel knew to follow her and bring her safely home. When Mom wanted to eat something, Rachel helped her navigate the kitchen. Both Daddy and I felt relieved that Mom was with a caring companion.

At first, Mom would forget who Rachel was as soon as Rachel left the house. Daddy and I made a point of referring to her as "your friend Rachel."

"Your friend Rachel is coming to visit tomorrow," I'd say in our phone conversations, but Mom still vociferously claimed she didn't need taking care of, and often she was in a bad mood when Rachel arrived. Rachel worked hard to dispel her moods as quickly as she could, and soon Mom was also referring to her as "my friend Rachel."

Weeks and months passed without incident. Then one Saturday night I got a call that Daddy was in the hospital. He'd driven himself—and Mom—there at four a.m. on Saturday morning, worried by his high blood pressure and a strong pain in his left shoulder. Sometime during the day they had managed to reach Rachel who had collected Mom from the hospital and stayed with her at my parents' home. There was nothing I could do right then, but I made my way straight to the hospital on Sunday morning as soon as it was light where I met up with Mom and Rachel who had also gone back that morning to see my dad. We learned that it was a false alarm: Daddy did not have a heart condition. Relieved, I sent Rachel home to get some sleep, and Mom and I drove back to their apartment.

By the time Daddy was released two days later, I was a wreck. I had been with Mom for forty-eight hours straight, and I needed a break. It was my first experience of being with Mom on a 24/7 basis. Not only had I neglected my own household, not to mention missing work, but I could not take a minute more of Mom's incessant questions regarding Daddy's whereabouts. I was tired of drinking tea. I was tired, too, of having no time to myself. I hated the way she followed me wherever I went. She'd stand close behind me while I typed on the computer. She even followed me to the bathroom.

I felt listless and used up. And I was angry at myself. I had come face to face with my inability to take care of Mom. What kind of daughter was I if I ran away at the first sign of stress? Should I expect more of myself? Or should I acknowledge my limitations? How did Daddy manage? If before I had given Daddy advice on how to remain calm in the face of Mom's irrational behavior, now I better understood his endless frustration.

Daddy listened to my heartache when I told him I felt like a lousy daughter for not being able to care for Mom. I got sympathy from friends, but Daddy was the one who could truly understand how I felt. He calmed me down. My primary role, he said, was to be the loving daughter whose presence Mom craved with increasing intensity. I vowed to be better at being with her.

Excellent and capable as Rachel was, more help would clearly be needed sooner than later. Daddy was urged by my parents' physician to be prepared, and to apply to the Israeli National Insurance Institute for permission to hire a full-time live-in caregiver. The process involved an initial assessment by a local social worker and presentation of medical documents asserting that Mom had Alzheimer's. If approved, the government would then kick in a large percentage of the monthly payments for a twenty-four-hour foreign worker. Since requests were often rejected the first time around and could take months for approval, it would be better to start the application process early so that we'd have the permission in hand when we really needed it.

The day the social worker arrived for the assessment, Mom was in great shape—a little too great, regrettably. While only the week before she'd been sure her son Simon was her cousin from England, this week she was more mentally acute. Daddy and I outlined the ways in which Mom was having difficulty, but when she got up from the table, went to the kitchen, and made tea for everyone, we knew we'd lost this round.

Three months later, Daddy managed on his own to convince the social worker that Mom needed assistance. The fact that Rachel was still coming every day to care for Mom was a factor in their favor. And when Mom couldn't remember the year or month, this too was a point. Permission to employ a full-time caregiver was received, with a time period of up to two years to actualize the hiring.

Realizing that Daddy needed help almost as much as Mom, that the house chores in addition to caring for Mom were too much for him, and that my visits, though they would continue, accounted for just a fraction of hours each week, Daddy decided it was time to hire someone. It was the end of 2013. We were three years into this disease, trying to cope daily with the unexpected and the inexplicable.

We were lucky to find Sahlee. As with hundreds of other Philippine caregivers, Sahlee had left her son in the care of her mother to work in Israel. The salary was higher in this type of work than anything Sahlee might earn inside the Philippines, and despite the large sum of money required to procure a work-in-Israel license, Sahlee was able to send money home each month to her family.

Sahlee took over the many day-to-day chores of running my parents' home. She did the laundry, changed sheets on the beds, got clothes out for Mom each day, washed the dishes, and even cooked. When I visited on Tuesdays, Sahlee often came with us to shop or drink coffee. She learned my parent's likes and dislikes, their routines, and ably assisted them.

Yet for all this, Mom was hostile toward Sahlee. She wouldn't let Sahlee help her shower or dress, and she got mad at her when she saw Sahlee usurping what used to be her rightful place in the kitchen. Daddy told her that Sahlee was there for him not her, and that at their age, it was nice to be taken care of. That worked some of the time.

One area in which Sahlee could not connect with Mom was on a cultural level. She had never heard most of the songs that Mom loved to sing or seen the movies that marked Mom's long-ago life. For this reason, we kept Rachel in our lives.

With Rachel caring for Mom one morning a week, a weekly Monday music concert, and my Tuesday visits, there was enough variety to engage Mom on many different levels.

* espe*

Visiting Mom on a weekly basis was not without stress. I worked hard to cook meals in advance for my family for when I arrived home after my long day of traveling. And if events in my community fell on a Tuesday, I often missed them as I was exhausted by the time I came home. I did, however, find myself in the kitchen cooking up batches of what I loved most.

There are some foods that are comforting in times of stress. For me, anything chocolate does the trick. I often hide chocolate bars around the house for emergency use. And if I team up my chocolate passion with peanut butter, that's a win-win basis for the ultimate treat. Here are two chocolate peanut butter cake recipes, one more hands-on than the other, but both equally good at satisfying my sweet-tooth and my stress.

Peanut Butter Chocolate Cheesecake

I make this cheesecake for the holiday of Shavuot. I make it only once a year—not because it's too complicated but because it is so good that I can't stop eating it. Don't have a blender? Crush cookies by placing them in a sealed bag and rolling with a rolling pin. Melt butter and chocolate together in the microwave and add to crushed cookies to form a chocolaty "dough." Don't forget to lick the bowl after spooning the filling onto the crust.

Crust:
1¾ cup petite beurre or other cookies, crushed or ground
6 Tbsp butter, melted
½ (or more) 100 gr / 3.5 oz bar of chocolate, crushed

Filling:
1 cup plain cream cheese (can be as low as 5%)
1 cup peanut butter
1 cup powdered sugar
1 tsp vanilla
½ cup whipping cream

Topping:
½ cup whipping cream
6 oz. / 170 gr semi-sweet chocolate chips

Directions:
In a food processor, mince cookies and chocolate. Melt butter in microwave for forty seconds and mix with minced cookies to form a "dough." Pat into nine-inch/twenty-three cm pie pan. In separate bowl, mix together the filling of cream cheese, peanut butter, sugar, and vanilla. Whip half the whipping cream with hand-held blender and fold into filling. Pour into the pie pan

and place in freezer. In microwave-safe bowl, pour in remaining whipping cream and add chocolate. Microwave for forty seconds, stir. Return to microwave for an additional forty seconds if chocolate is not melted. Remove pie from freezer and pour microwaved cream on top. Return to freezer. Defrost before serving.

Peanut Butter Chocolate Swirl Cake[7]

What can I say? This cake batter is so good you might find yourself eating it raw. Don't worry too much if that happens. No one will be able to tell.

½ cup peanut butter
⅓ cup oil
1 cup sugar
½ cup brown sugar
2 eggs
1 tsp vanilla
1 cup flour
1 tsp baking powder
½ tsp salt
Chocolate chips (enough to cover top of cake)

Directions:
Mix oil, sugars and peanut butter. Add eggs and vanilla. Mix in dry ingredients. When batter is formed, pat into greased eight-inch / twenty-cm round pan or English cake pan then sprinkle with chocolate chips. Push chips gently into batter. Use enough chips to cover top of cake. Bake at 350 degrees F / 180 degrees C for 5 minutes. Remove pan from oven and using a knife, pull some of the peanut butter batter up from underneath the chocolate to give the cake a swirl pattern. Clean knife carefully with your tongue. Return pan to oven and bake for an additional thirty minutes.

---

[7] Based on a recipe in *Modiin Cuisine,* compiled by Freda and Yoni Bak

Alzheimer's Pantoum

"How are you today?" she asks
as if it's the first time. I tell her
I'm fine, I'm taking a poetry class,
Liora's got a solo in the school musical.

As if it's the first time, I tell her
we're all fine. Hillel made a new friend,
Liora's got a solo in the school musical.
"How are you today?" she asks.

We're all fine! Hillel made a new friend.
We chatter away about small things.
"How are you today?" she asks.
It's cold outside, and she's dressed for summer.

We chatter away about small things.
I thought she'd always be my mother.
It's snowing outside, and she's dressed for summer.
Her mind keeps its secrets.

I thought she'd always be my mother.
Now my skills exceed hers.
Her mind keeps its secrets,
memory as cruel as winter.

Now my skills exceed hers.
"How are you today?" she asks,
memory as cruel as winter.
I'm fine, I'm taking a poetry class.

after Linda Pastan

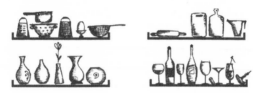

Chapter 5

Grapefruit Sandwiches and Other Quirks

I dream about you," Mom said to me one morning. We were sitting together on the couch in her living room. "Oh, really? What do you dream?" I asked.

"I dream you are with me, and when I wake up, I can't remember if you're here or not."

"That must be hard to sort out," I said, trying for empathy and understanding.

"You don't know the half of it," she replied.

The summer I was sixteen, I was part of a program that tried to physically show us what it was like to grow old. We wore glasses with Vaseline smeared on the lenses to limit our vision, plugged our ears with cotton to distort sound, and tied thick blocks to our shoes to unbalance us. The effect was unnerving, as if only half our senses were working. We treated it like a game, after all, we were young and invincible.

I tried to keep those unbalanced feelings in mind when I visited Mom.

Mom was constantly confused by the sights, sounds, and conversations that swirled around her. She couldn't keep up with even the simplest of arrangements. If Daddy had chores to do, Mom asked again and again where he was going. If he said he'd be back shortly, she started to panic. If he left without her, she accused him of abandoning her. "You're dumping me here," she cried. Nothing about her days was normal.

"Normal is just a setting on your dryer," said a friend who was a social worker.

When I recounted some of the funny things Mom had done, like hiding her handbag under her pillow or making a sandwich with humus and grapefruit slices, this woman, who works with Alzheimer's and dementia patients, reiterated that caring for someone with Alzheimer's meant throwing our definitions of "normal" out the window.

When I was with Mom, my task was to keep her on a regular schedule of activities, get her to places on time, help her interact with family and friends—in short, assist her in conforming to expected behaviors.

What happened when Mom's schedule and her behaviors clashed? How crucial was it for Mom to "fit in" with the rest of the world? The test was finding my creativity in the face of Mom's emotional quirks and derailments.

Mom's instinct for social interaction was incredibly strong. When we were out on the streets of the city, we often paused in our ramblings to say hello to people she knew. Sometimes, though, it was random strangers who were the targets of her sincere and infectious cheerfulness.

When we stopped in a jewelry store to see the displays, Mom enthusiastically greeted a woman at the counter as an old friend.

"Do I know you?" the woman asked Mom.

"It's been a long time since we've seen each other," Mom replied.

The woman was obviously confused. I didn't want to blurt out to this stranger that Mom had Alzheimer's. Mom would probably be insulted and deny it. And by labeling Mom, I would be limiting the way this woman viewed her. The more Mom interacted, though, the easier it was for most people to figure out that something was not quite right, especially as her sentences became illogical.

I was conscious of standing outside the unfolding encounter, but unlike how my kids probably felt when I embarrassed them, I knew it was useless being embarrassed by Mom's behavior. I couldn't control how she interacted with the world, nor would I want to. I could only guide her and keep her safe.

"I think we've made a mistake," I finally said, stepping in to take Mom's hand and lead her out. "But it is a pleasure to meet friendly people with nice smiles."

The woman visibly relaxed, and Mom, as a parting gift, gave her a big hug.

When she made her grapefruit and humus sandwich, I quickly diverted her from eating it, explaining that it probably wouldn't taste good. The rind was still on the grapefruit slices, and if she had been in her right mind, she would not have made it, let alone fought me to eat it.

The issue, though, is that it *was* her "right mind." Mom has only one mind, and by definition it is the right one, regardless of her perception of reality.

Maybe the burden lay with me. Did I have the power to creatively change the situation? Instead of scolding her for doing something foolish, which was often my first response, could I point out in a humorous way that grapefruits taste better on their own? Or give her the tools to fix her sandwich by offering her something different to eat with her humus?

It takes an extraordinary stable temperament to deal with an Alzheimer's patient on a daily basis. Getting them up and dressed in the morning can be filled with hurdles. Sometimes Mom puts her shirt on inside out or wears a thick sweater in the middle of summer. Or she forgets to brush her teeth. What works once to convince her to change might not work the next time. It is a constant game of give and take and trying new things.

Perhaps it's about how uncomfortable *we* are with the non-normative behavior of Alzheimer's patients. I can't see myself letting Mom eat a grapefruit humus sandwich. But the world won't stop if she refuses to brush her teeth. Our job is to take their lead and guide them to live with dignity, love, and happiness within societal norms. It can be pretty darn uncomfortable to wear your underwear backward.

c/ɔe/ɔ

The constant conflict between typical behavior and Mom's atypical outbursts pushed me to reevaluate the way I treated her. It was a catalyst for my self-improvement.

On a beautiful Monday in spring of 2015, Daddy happened to be in Jerusalem on a day I was also there. He picked me up and we made our way back to Netanya after our separate conferences were over. I would stay the night and then devote my usual Tuesday to Mom.

It was rare for Daddy to spend a whole day away from Mom. He knew how anxious she got when he was not with her. In the past, he had asked me to cover for him if he would be away for a period of more than several hours. This time, I hadn't been available. I called from the car to tell Mom—and alert her caregiver Sahlee—that we'd be arriving in about half an hour. I could hear Mom's panicked voice on the phone.

"I'll be with the dead people."

"What?" I asked into the phone. "What did you say?"

"I'll be with the dead people," Mom repeated.

I wanted to ask what she meant, but I knew Mom couldn't explain the isolation and abandonment she was experiencing. I started saying anything that might calm her. I even tried singing on the phone, hoping she'd sing along.

"Why don't you have a cup of tea and a biscuit?" I finally suggested, appealing to her British nature. "We'll be home in about twenty minutes."

"I can't open the door and I want to go home," she cried. "This is not my home. Where's Jack?"

It took all of my wits to talk Mom down from the despair she was feeling. She was so upset at not having Daddy near her that she'd angrily told Sahlee that she needed to leave to go to her real home.

When we reached Netanya, we heard her through the door impatiently asking Sahlee to unlock it so that she could see her *father*. Standing in the hallway, Daddy and I shared that moment with an unspoken shrug: No matter how much we gave to Mom, we would often not be recognized by her for who we were. It lent new meaning to acting selflessly.

In fact, even after seeing Daddy and greeting him effusively, Mom insisted on going out. I barely had a chance to put my bags down before the two of us were outside in the bright afternoon. We walked to the promenade by the sea and sat on a bench in the shade. We watched the passersby, sang a few songs, and Mom visibly relaxed.

"I love that tufty soft earth," Mom said.

"Do you mean the grass?"

"Yes, and the wispy white up there."

"The clouds."

"Yes. And the way the water sparkles in the sun."

A half hour later, we went back to the apartment.

Nothing could have equipped us for Mom's emotional response to Daddy's absence. The episodic nature of Alzheimer's meant that we had to be prepared for anything, and we had to think fast. This visit had demanded my most considerate self. I entered her world as best I could and gave to her as if she were my precious child. That's what she needed. Mom was teaching me through her Alzheimer's the enormity of what it meant to honor my parents.

೧ು೧

One of the pleasures of making soup is the minimum amount of time it takes to pull it all together. A side benefit of making it with Mom was that when she was first diagnosed, Mom was still able to help cut vegetables. Once I reminded her how to cube, slice, or chop, she was part of the process, too. It felt almost like old times, together in the kitchen.

As queen of the kitchen, Mom was the traditional soup maker in the family when I was growing up. Often, Mom would use pre-packaged soup ingredients to make dinner when she had little time to prepare. *Streit's* soup packages were the perfect solution for the working woman who wanted to give her family a healthy meal, especially on cold winter evenings. The ingredients were in a see-through package that was a little wider than my closed fist and the layers of lentils, barley, other legumes, and spices formed a colorful three-dimensional roll that rattled when I shook it. It amazed me how the disparate parts could form a tasty, nutritious whole in the soup Mom served.

If she arrived home late from work, Mom would use her pressure cooker to speed up the soup's progress. I vividly recall the horrible moan as steam gushed from her pressure cooker. "Stand back!" she'd instruct and rush forward to cap the vent with the regulator. I hated that pot. I was afraid the steam would burn her as she balanced the regulator on a fork tong over the vent. I imagined the whole lid coming loose and popping off from the strong rush of steam. I swore never to use one. Today the pressure cooker sits silent in the back of Mom's kitchen cupboard. When I make soup, I use fresh ingredients and make sure I have enough time to let it cook to a gradual perfection.

Orange Soup

The appearance of orange soup in our house means that winter is fast approaching. This rich-bodied soup is a combination of fall vegetables: carrots, pumpkin, and sweet potato. To make it a complete meal, we add a cup of red lentils. If you want a lighter soup to eat as a first course, leave out the lentils.

1 large onion, chopped
3 cloves garlic, crushed
1 cup red lentils
1 large sweet potato, chopped
4-5 carrots, chopped
½ lb / ¼ kilo (about 1 cup) orange pumpkin, chopped
2 tsp dried basil or 2-3 sprigs fresh basil, chopped
3-4 sprigs fresh parsley, chopped
1 small parsley root, peeled and chopped
Salt and pepper to taste
Water to cover (approximately 6 to 8 cups)

Directions:
In a large pot, sauté onions and garlic. Add lentils and sauté for a few more minutes. Add chopped vegetables and cover with water. (Additional water will make a thinner soup.) Add spices. Bring to a boil, then simmer for up to an hour or until vegetables are soft. Using a hand-held blender, blend the remaining soup right in the pot. Can be served hot or cold.

Lentil Mushroom Soup

My husband Jeff is our family's soup-maker extraordinaire. His chicken soup is a dark mix of finely chopped vegetables and spices that explodes with taste. And you should try his matza balls! He has allowed me to share this "secret" recipe for lentil soup that he formulated after several trials, which we all ate enthusiastically. There is a subtle earthy taste to this thick textured soup. So good you'll want seconds.

4 cups red lentils
4-5 cups mushrooms, sliced (preferably porcini, but button mushrooms work, too)
1 19-oz / 550-gr can pre-cooked chickpeas, drained
2 onions, chopped
3 carrots, chopped
6-8 cloves garlic, minced
2 Tbsp brown sugar
3-4 bay leaves
½ tsp dried basil
½ tsp dried oregano
Pinch of thyme
Salt and coarse black pepper to taste
Water as specified in directions

Directions:
In a large pot, cook mushrooms in 4 cups water. Let cool and puree in a blender along with garbanzo beans. Return to pot. Add remaining ingredients plus an additional 4-6 cups water. Bring to a boil then simmer for up to 4 hours (or more) stirring occasionally.

Kitchen Sink Soup

When the kids ask me what's in the soup, I reply like Mom taught me: "Everything but the kitchen sink." I make variations of this soup all the time, depending on what I have in the house. It's a relatively easy recipe to follow. The basics are a can of crushed tomatoes, a plentiful amount of vegetables, and a cup of lentils. I've been known to add cabbage, spinach, broccoli, even peas. Enjoy it on a cold winter night.

2 Tbsp olive oil
1 onion, chopped
4 cloves garlic, crushed
2 carrots, diced
3 stalks celery, diced (with leaves)
1 cup pumpkin, chopped
½ cup fresh parsley, chopped
1 tsp dried oregano
1 tsp dried basil
2-3 bay leaves
1 800 gr / 28 oz can crushed tomatoes
1 cup green lentils
½ cup barley or brown rice (optional)
6 to 8 cups water
Salt and pepper to taste

Directions:
In a large pot, sauté onions and garlic in olive oil until onions become translucent. Add vegetables and spices. Cook an additional five minutes. Add the lentils and barley (if using). Add water. Bring soup to a boil, then cover and simmer on low heat for at least an hour.

Cauliflower Soup

Sometimes, the easier a dish, the better. Here's a summer soup that takes so little effort and produces a creamy taste sensation, all with only three ingredients (if you don't count the water)—cauliflower, onion and garlic. Serve it cold on hot summer evenings. Or serve it delight-fully warm. This recipe, using two cauliflower heads, is enough for eight servings.

2 heads cauliflower, cleaned and chopped into florets
1 large onion, chopped
3-4 garlic cloves, chopped
6 cups water
Salt and pepper to taste

Directions:
Sauté garlic and onions in a large pot until onions become translucent. Add in cauliflower and cover in water. Stir in salt and pepper. (Make sure you add enough salt as cauliflower can be bland.) Bring to a boil then simmer for thirty minutes until cauliflower is soft. Remove water and save in a different container. Using a hand-held blender, blend cauliflower until creamy, adding back water until the soup is the consistency you like, either thick or thin. Serve with chopped scallions and soup nuts. Note: Frozen cauliflower works, too!

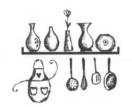
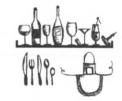

The Slow Escape

This is the part where she curls in on herself
in a slow, fragile dance,
a nightly performance
for an audience of one or two,
rabbits pulling her out of their hats,
something clearly up their sleeves.
Houdini locked himself in a milk can
with a hidden hollow space
so he could breathe
while he picked the locks.
Her routine uses no trick handcuffs,
no illusions.
This disease knows all the secrets, anyway.
Pay close attention.
This is the hardest act yet.
The main actor
does an imitation
of my mother
as she smiles and laughs
and lulls me with her patter,
fading into a nothingness
even the Great Magician could not escape.

Chapter 6

Balancing the Scales

As harsh as it sounds, I have learned to use Mom's Alzheimer's for my own needs. I wasn't necessarily proud of my behavior or the way it reflected on me, but it helped me on several levels—my need to preserve an essence of Mom and easing Mom's stubbornness over some task or other.

When it came to savoring Mom's essence, I started telling friends that the jewelry I wore or the bowl gracing my table had been "liberated" from Mom's house.

The first time? I stole a shirt from Mom's drawer. Or maybe I borrowed it permanently. Did the nuance in the confession ameliorate my guilt?

It happened so innocently. As we were getting ready to leave the house, Daddy noticed that Mom was wearing two skirts.

"How did that happen?" Mom wondered.

"They must have been stuck together," I suggested, trying to spin it positively.

"Yesterday you had on two shirts," Daddy said, chuckling. "Maybe you're balancing the scales today."

Mom laughed too. She started taking off the outer skirt, but it was tight around her waist. We couldn't figure out how she'd put it on. Mom didn't realize how much weight she had gained. Whereas she used to eat small portions and refuse most cakes, these days she was eating with abandon, sometimes forgetting that she'd just had a full meal.

We pulled the skirt up over her head and went into the bedroom to put it away.

Mom opened her drawer rather than her closet and became distracted. "What's this?" she asked, holding up a white and green top. "Is this a bathing suit?"

"No," I said, eyeing it with interest. "It's the same kind of material, but you wear this over another shirt, like a jumper."

"Oh," she replied.

I don't remember Mom ever wearing this shirt. I noticed how elegantly the neck fell in folds from a small weight sewn into the extra material.

"Here, I'll take it," I said. Then I closed the drawer, hung the skirt in the closet, and gathered Mom to go out. Along the way, I slipped that shirt into my knapsack.

Like taking candy from a baby. She had no awareness of my stealth and there was no chance that she'd remember it.

In 2014, we culled a lot of clothes from her overstuffed wardrobe that Mom never wore. Our goal was to make room in the closet for the clothes she did wear, leaving a wide range of options for her to choose from. We had to do it in secret, because each item I took from the closet she'd grab back and say, "Don't take that, I wear it all the time." It was useless to argue with her. Some of the clothes hadn't been worn in decades.

There was a scene in the movie *Sideways* where Paul Giamatti's character stole money from his mom's purse while she was sleeping. I didn't like the movie, and I definitely didn't like that scene. I would never condone theft and certainly not from the elderly.

Judaism regards stealing in secret as a more heinous crime than stealing openly. If you openly steal something, you show a disregard for the opinion and rights of others. If you steal secretly, you are acting hypocritically, because you understand the consequences of your actions; you are afraid of the opinion of others yet disregard what God thinks and steal nonetheless.

I did feel guilty. I took advantage of the simple nature that Alzheimer's had bequeathed my Mom for my own benefit, even if I knew it didn't hurt her.

On the other hand, every time I wear that shirt, I think of Mom. I feel her close to me, as if she is giving me one of her special hugs. To me, that balances the scales.

෴

Could I really justify manipulating Mom through her memory loss?

Every year when Mom's birthday rolled around, I was struck not only by another year passing, but by the idea that there was almost nothing I could give her as a gift.

What kind of present could I buy for the person whose needs were shrinking? She barely wore jewelry anymore, just the same favorite earrings and necklace. She didn't read. She didn't cook. She didn't travel. She didn't buy new clothes. She didn't even enjoy eating out anymore. (By the time the meal arrived, Mom couldn't remember having ordered it, and she ate so slowly, she was better off at home.) When I thought back to how capable Mom was just a few years ago, I realized how much of her we had lost.

"To forget your birthday is…tragic," Mom declared in a moment of clarity. We watched her bounce between unbridled joy, disbelief, and even annoyance as she "discovered" it was her seventy-fifth birthday.

The first time we told her, she expressed such enthusiasm.

"It is?" she asked in a child-like voice.

The third time, she rebuked me.

"Don't be ridiculous," she said. "I don't have time for that nonsense."

Birthdays were always fun occasions when I was growing up. For one of my birthdays, I remember my friends being blind-folded and led one-by-one through a maze in our basement. When the blind-fold was removed, the maze had disappeared. All our jumps, all the exhortations to step to the left or right, were pretend. I marveled at the cleverness of my parents to invent this fun game, especially as, once we'd been through the "maze," we encouraged our friends from the sidelines and watched as they exerted themselves.

How strange that this was the memory that surfaced; Mom navigated daily the maze of her mind's making.

By the time we'd left for a birthday lunch at a nearby restaurant, Mom was enchanted again.

When she turned seventy-three, we had given Mom a mug with a photo of the family on it. For her seventy-fourth, the gift that I put together was a wall frame with eight photos of our immediate family that I dutifully labeled with everyone's names. Mom loved it. But as I gave it to her, I realized my phone wasn't recording her wondrous reaction. Thinking quickly, I took back the gift, waited ten minutes, and presented it to her again, this time with the camera rolling. The same beautiful smiles at seeing all her loved ones was now recorded.

I was both amused and horrified by my use of Mom's Alzheimer's. It was a trick I tried not to employ too often, but it worked when I needed Mom to do something, like swallowing her pills, or taking off her coat, things she was reticent to do. If she wouldn't acquiesce the first time, she might the second...or perhaps the seventh.

I kept reminding myself to think positively. Mom was happy. She laughed and sang. She told jokes. She clapped along to music. She enjoyed taking walks. She was engaged in the now.

Mom received several birthday cards in honor of her seventy-fifth birthday which she puzzled over. The one that excited her the most was from her sister, Barbara in England. It read, "Happy birthday, sister..." Mom wanted to use the card to call Barbara.

At the restaurant for her birthday lunch, we surreptitiously asked the waitress to bring us a dessert with a sparkler. Mom was excited. Then, when the sparkler was placed in front of her on the table, she became frightened and insisted we remove it. Her mood spoiled and she wouldn't even eat any of the cake.

As we walked back, Mom didn't recognize any of the streets near her house.

"I've never been this way before," she said.

And at the apartment door, she hesitated going inside what she thought was someone else's home. We had to gently convince her at each step that she was in the right place.

When she woke from her nap, Mom had another surprise waiting. Her caregiver, Sahlee, had made her a cake.

"It's my birthday?" she asked innocently.

She loved the lit candles and happily made a wish as she blew them out.

Perhaps the best "present" we could give Mom was to be with her in the present. As my husband Jeff told each of our kids, "It may seem pointless to call and wish her a happy birthday since she doesn't really know who we are—and won't remember a minute later. But for that moment, it has tremendous value."

Finding the joy in the day was a gift not to be wasted, especially on her birthday.

My wish for Mom was to have a year of being loved for who she was and who she is becoming, a year of comfort as her mind and body continued to disintegrate.

ℰↃℰↃ

What sealed birthdays when I was young were the cakes Mom used to make. My mouth still waters when I think of them: airy profusions of yellow cake with cinnamon topping, or gooey chocolate syrup cakes. But my all-time favorites were the "failure cakes." That's what we called them. Dense, moist batter that rose to underdone perfection, a rich, wine-soaked cake with a hint of nutmeg. They were anything but failures in our eyes.

I can't remember why she let us eat the first one. Had she left out an ingredient? Or misjudged the cooking time? Maybe my brother and I were the culprits. We'd already had one fire in the house due to our fighting. Simon and I had been in the basement doing our usual thing—annoying each other. He usually got the better of me, despite being younger, and it was all I could do to manipulate my parents into thinking it was his fault, even when it clearly wasn't. This time, the noise of our argument had become so heated that Mom came downstairs to pull us apart. We were still following her back up the stairs when we heard her scream. Flames from the pot on the stove were spreading across the ceiling, and smoke filled the kitchen stretching in thick roiling waves through the hallway. Overcoming her utter fear, Mom doused the flames by putting the lid on the pot, then grabbed the extinguisher and quenched the blaze before it consumed the entire kitchen. At least she got a new range out of that disaster.

Whatever the case, Mom's failure cakes were delicious; we always begged her to make more. And she kept making those cakes especially for us. The flaw became perfection.

Failure cakes are an apt metaphor for Alzheimer's. What have I learned in turning this disease on its head, in finding a kind of success within the failure?

How challenging it is to see Mom's behavior—the life she lives with its many limitations—as positive. We are constantly aware that, sooner or later, Alzheimer's will claim all of Mom. Thinking about the future, I couldn't always keep my emotions in check. In my darker moments, I cried for the loss of my beloved mother.

But I also achingly accepted her replacement, the sweet simple woman who had trouble remembering who I was. Though it was always new for her, for me, my weekly visits with Mom held a pattern, a semblance of a routine of place and activity. It didn't matter how many times we drank coffee in the same café, or window shopped in the same stores. What mattered was that we were together. We enjoyed ourselves. I loved those moments of absolute joy and laughter as much as she did.

When I think back to those awesome cakes, none of us remembered a specific recipe for "failure" cake. When my kids were growing up, we made an assortment of birthday cakes, mainly chocolate or vanilla-flavored in different shapes, the most impressive being a train or a doll in a skirt, Winnie the Pooh, Spiderman and Batman. Now that they have grown, "crumble cake" is the optimal favorite as it combines chocolate and vanilla, has a pleasing, moist consistency and a soft cinnamon-flavored crumble topping.

When I looked through the recipes Mom had sent me when we moved to Israel, there was one marked, "The Cake." Though my kids gave it mixed reviews, its wine-sweetened batter bursting with nutmeg took me back to my childhood and still does whenever I make it.

These cakes can be made easily by hand with a fork and a mixing bowl, or you can also use an electric mixer or beater. Essential items for cake making: measuring cups for both liquid and dry ingredients, and measuring spoons. Also have on hand a variety of baking pans, either square, round or Bundt (that's the one with the hole in the middle). These cakes can all be baked at 350 degrees F / 180 degrees C. For converting measurements, use these formulas:

3 Tbsp = ¼ cup = 2 oz. = 50 grams.
1 cup = 8 oz. = 200 grams

The Cake

The sophisticated taste and moist batter yield an elegant cake that's a treat for guests. Or keep it for yourself, because you can.

½ cup vegetable oil
1 cup sugar
4 eggs
2 tsp baking powder
¾ cup sherry or dry red wine
1 tsp nutmeg
2 cups flour
1 2.8 oz / 80 gr pkg instant vanilla pudding

Directions:
Beat eggs and sugar, then whisk in oil. Add sherry and remaining ingredients and mix thoroughly. Bake in a greased Bundt pan for thirty-five minutes at 350 degrees F / 180 degrees C.

Crumble Cake

This cake always appeases my kids' disparate requests for vanilla vs. chocolate-flavored cakes. The batter is enough to fill two small eight-inch/twenty-cm pans or one large pan ten-inch / twenty-five-cm.

¾ cup canola oil
2 cups sugar
4 cups flour
4 tsp baking powder
½ tsp salt
1½ cup milk (or milk-substitute, i.e., soy milk or orange juice)
1½ tsp vanilla
2 eggs
½ to ¼ cup cocoa powder
1½ tsp cinnamon

Directions:
In a small bowl, beat oil and sugar then add remaining dry ingredients. Set aside 1 cupful for the crumble topping. Add egg, vanilla and milk (or milk substitute) to the dry ingredients and mix well. Divide batter. In one bowl, add cocoa powder. To create a marble effect, pour alternating layers of vanilla and chocolate batter into a baking pan. Gently swirl a knife or spatula through the batter. Add cinnamon to cup mixture that was set aside and crumble on top. Bake at 350 degrees F / 180 degrees C for approximately forty minutes.

Deep Dark Chocolate Cake

Though the number of ingredients may seem imposing, this is a cake that works even if you "schittareyn," as my grandmother would say (Yiddish for "pour it all in together").

2 cups flour
1½ cups sugar
1 cup cocoa
1½ tsp baking powder
1½ tsp baking soda
1 tsp vanilla
2 eggs
½ cup canola oil
1 cup milk or ½ cup orange juice and ½ cup water
1 cup hot water

Icing:
½ cup chocolate chips
1 tsp vanilla
1 tsp water

Directions:
Preheat oven to 350 degrees F / 180 degrees C. Measure dry ingredients into a bowl and mix. Add oil, vanilla, eggs and milk or orange juice and water and continue mixing batter. Add hot water last: heat one cup of water in the microwave for sixty seconds. Slowly work it into the batter. Pour into greased pan ten-inch / twenty-five cm and bake for forty-five to fifty minutes. To prepare icing, measure chips, water and vanilla and heat on high for forty seconds in a microwave-safe measuring cup. Stir and repeat until chips are melted. Pour over cooling cake.

Lemon Bars

I was given this recipe at my bridal shower and I still make it 28 years later. I remember walking in the door to my parent's home and being utterly surprised by the gathering there of friends and family. Mom outdid herself in the fancy spread of salads and dessert.

Crust:
2 cups flour
½ cup canola oil
½ cup powdered sugar

Filling:
4 eggs
2 cups sugar
6 Tbsp lemon juice
¼ cup flour
½ tsp baking powder

Directions:
Mix crust ingredients together. Pat into nine-inch / twenty-three-cm pan and bake for fifteen minutes at 350 degrees F / 180 degrees C. In a separate bowl, mix eggs, sugar, lemon juice and remaining ingredients. Pour over cooled crust and bake for an additional fifteen to twenty minutes. When cooled, sprinkle with powdered sugar.

Mud Pie

This recipe is adapted from my signed copy of the Kosher Southern-Style Cookbook *(Pelican Publishing Co., 1993) that I received from my mother-in-law. I couldn't find corn syrup in Israel, so I started using maple-flavored pancake syrup as a substitute. It came out so well, I continued using it even when corn syrup finally showed up in my grocery store.*

Crust:
1½ cups flour
½ cup canola oil
5 Tbsp cold water
1 tsp salt
pinch of sugar

Filling:
⅓ Canola oil
1 cup sugar
3 eggs
3 Tbsp maple-flavored pancake syrup (or corn syrup)
1 tsp vanilla
1 tsp water
½ cup (or more) chocolate chips

Directions:
Mix crust ingredients and pat into round nine-inch / twenty-three-cm pie pan. In a large bowl, mix eggs, oil, sugar and syrup. In a glass measuring cup, measure water, vanilla and chips. Melt in microwave on high for 40 seconds, more if needed. Stir until chips are melted. Blend melted chocolate with eggs mixture. Pour filling into crust and bake at 350 degrees F / 180 degrees C for thirty to forty minutes or until top is slightly brittle.

Solitary

When the storm
turns and says in my mother's voice
I am solitary next to you,

I think these things:

She is two-thirds empty and one-third confusion.
And the two-thirds are her past and her future.

Or maybe its three-fourths exhaustion.
Or perhaps she is an instrument of God.

When the storm turns cold
and says in my mother's voice
I am solitary next to you,

I remember these things:

A mother's love
is bananas and sugar mashed in milk,
one cup worry, a pinch of grief, and what's left over
sweetens the scones and conversation we shared.

And dreaming? Behind her drooping eyes
is a place that is whole.

And loving? She kisses me
as if I've been away for years.

When storm that rattles my windows says
I am solitary next to you,

I know it's me
or my mother through me, asking,

Can you handle this loss?
Will you forgive yourself if you break?

Strange. A misplaced mother.
A storm with a voice.
And my heart talking to God.

after Li-young Lee

Chapter 7

Sundowning and Other Symptoms

The photos on Mom's dresser hadn't changed in years. There was an engagement photo of me and my brother with our respective spouses the summer we both got engaged, one of my oldest as a baby—Mom's first grandson (who now has a child of his own), and a flattering photo of me when I turned twenty-one. I was pleased that the photos were still on her dresser.

We were in Mom's room organizing the clothes in her dresser drawers. Each week during my visit, we'd sort and fold the clothes in Mom's drawers because in the intervening days, clothes that didn't belong and other items would make their way in there. It was important to me that Mom have access to her clothes so that she could make choices about what to wear; but keeping items in their place was difficult for her. It also allowed me to surreptitiously cull the clothes that no longer fit her or that she did not wear. On one occasion, I struggled to open the middle drawer that I knew held T-shirts to find three big heavy sweaters shoved in there. Another time, we solved the puzzle of Mom's lost glasses when we found them at the bottom of her underwear drawer. When Sahlee started working for them, my parents' house became tidier.

"That's me," I said, seeing my former self as a young woman.

That summer we were in London visiting family and we'd gone out to celebrate in a posh restaurant with my aunt, uncle, cousins, and some close family friends. I was about to start my Oberlin-in-London semester abroad, reading and watching plays in London's theaters, and wandering around my birth city as a single, unencumbered young woman. The world held exciting possibilities.

"That's a lovely photo," Mom replied. "Does your mom have a copy?"

Huh? My head swiveled round so quickly, I felt dizzy. Mom was standing next to me absorbed in the photos. She was calm, unperturbed. She didn't realize that she'd just erased our shared past.

"Well, yes, she does," I managed to squeak out.

And there it ended. We moved on to other things, other topics, planning our day together, songs we should sing, perhaps a walk in the park.

Sometimes I couldn't get used to all I'd lost. There was a terrible emotional strain to realizing that Mom could no longer comfort me as a parent comforts a child, as I yearned to be comforted. Often we'd be singing a song together from my childhood, my croaky frog pipes beside her melodious voice, and I'd start to cry, choking back the tears so as not to alarm Mom, because the song would bring up exactly the emotions I was trying so hard not to feel. Then reality interceded and I had to become a caregiver and put aside my role of daughter.

In addition to robbing her of her memories, Alzheimer's had pilfered other abilities from Mom, foremost her ability to understand reality. Some of the malevolent symptoms that I'd discovered while taking care of her were surprising and confusing not only to Mom, but to me as well.

There are a group of behaviors such as increased anxiety, pacing, paranoia and volatile anger that sometimes peak in Alzheimer's patients as the sun goes down. Sundowning, or late day confusion, affects individuals at a specific time of day. Mom would be relatively fine, often being the most lucid in the mornings, when all of a sudden, as the sun descended, she exhibited unpredictable behaviour.

Mom's apartment has a large bank of windows in the living room. It was easy to track the sun's descent from these windows, the long shadows that crept in on early winter evenings, and the bright, blasting sun that shone down during the summer. In summer, Mom might wake from a nap to several more hours of light and wish us all "good morning." We made sure to keep the shutters at an angle during the hottest part of the day, but as the sun made it's descent, and an orange glow filtered into the apartment, we turned on the lights in the living room and opened the shutters to allow for more light to enter. This was one way of combatting Sundowning. Other ideas that seemed to help combat Sundowning were sticking to a schedule, and making sure Mom slept well but also kept active.

Researchers agree that Sundowning occurs during the day's transition from light to dark, but they do not know its cause. It remains as elusive as the cause of Alzheimer's itself.

When she was in the throes of looking for the way home, often as darkness descended, Mom had a tendency to wander through the house seeking something that was "lost." She'd open and close doors, enter and exit a room, move books from one shelf to another, or even remove random—and sometimes important—documents from closed file folders. She would also get herself into trouble. Once, she turned on the faucet and was shocked by the gushing water that splashed her full force. Fortunately, it was the cold tap as otherwise she could have been scalded. We tried to be prepared for the unexpected when the sun went down.

As strange as the notion that the setting sun affects people with dementia is the skill with which they carried on conversations as if their brains were not damaged. There is a verbal trick that people with Alzheimer's employ when they are stuck for words: they confabulate. In mid- to late-stages of the disease, memory loss and cognitive problems lead to confusion and contribute to false perceptions.

As Alzheimer's sufferers struggle to make sense of their surroundings—to remember objects or recognize faces—their minds construct fabrications to fill in the gaps they are experiencing. This is a form of confabulation, an unconscious distortion of reality or misinterpreted memories that often surface in chatty conversations with Mom.

When friends told me Mom sounded good, I agreed with them rather than expose the ways in which Mom really didn't make much sense. Mom had the ability to fool people with social niceties. She may not have known who she was talking to, but she remembered how to be polite, to answer in general terms that she was doing well and yesterday was so hot, and how are you? And if they asked her something she didn't understand, she'd switch the topic.

"You have a lovely smile," she'd say, gently touching the chin of her fellow conversationalist, "and you should be blessed with happiness."

My friends loved Mom's enthusiasm and the powerful, positive blessings she bestowed upon them.

Confabulation is accompanied by other forms of distorted reality that are associated with Alzheimer's. If you've spent any time with someone suffering from Alzheimer's, you know they talk in strange, often disconnected language. They misname things or speak in odd, rambling, disjointed sentences. They become agitated and swear with the foulest of language—a particularly big shock if they've been polite, reserved ladies or gentlemen all their lives.

Those who have Alzheimer's are unable to experience reality as it really is. They suffer from delusions and hallucinations, two pernicious symptoms bestowed upon them by the disease.

Delusions are false beliefs. Even if you try to convince your loved one that the cat can't really ride a bicycle, she won't change her belief. Delusions can be both positive and negative. Mom often put aside food on her plate because she was saving it for someone else. Or she was certain that Daddy was going to abandon her because he left the house for a meeting.

She was often suspicious even of those closest to her. She accused us—her caregivers—of locking her in the apartment when she needed to go "home," often because the light was fading or because there was a break in her routine.

The fact is that we did indeed lock a second upper deadbolt on the front door that we knew Mom couldn't unlock herself. This was to prevent her from leaving the apartment on her own as she had done in the past. Once, when Sahlee was away on her day off and my dad was in the shower, Mom let herself out of the apartment with

Daddy's keys and took his cell phone, too. When he realized she was gone, Daddy called the police. They tried to persuade him to wait at home. But he could not sit still. He set out by car to see if he could find her, knowing that if she realized she was lost, she would be incapable of finding her way home by herself. After searching for about twenty minutes, he returned home with a heavy heart, hoping that she would somehow also return. When the home phone rang, it was with great relief that Daddy learned that a friend had found Mom wandering in the city's main square and had taken her to his home.

Unfortunately, in this instance, Mom was not exaggerating or imagining it when she claimed that we locked her in the house.

Hallucinations are incorrect perceptions of objects or events involving the senses. What seems real to the person experiencing them cannot be verified by anyone else. Most often, these experiences involve visual or auditory hallucinations. They, too, can be both positive and negative, or even whimsical especially if they are memory-related. One afternoon, as she was brushing her hair, Mom started brushing my hair too, vividly recalling how as a child she would brush her grandmother's long hair. We had a whole conversation in which she talked to me as if I were her grandmother (for whom I'm named). They apparently lived in the same house until her grandmother's death. I cannot say for certain that what she related to me was actual. I remember her telling similar stories before she was ill, so I had some sense against which to measure the banter. I finally told her I had to use the toilet so as to end the whole strange scenario of me being confused for her grandmother.

More than once, Mom had told me that her young children were in the next room, and when she couldn't find them, she'd say that they must have gone out to play.

Hallucinations can involve smell and taste and even physical sensations. Medicines, including anti-anxiety pills that are often prescribed for Alzheimer's patients, sometimes trigger hallucinations.

It must be a lonely and isolating experience to navigate a constantly changing world where your perception of reality is faulty. Established, unambiguous principles and objects that I as a rational adult take for granted have no consistency for someone with Alzheimer's. Each day brings new and often frightening challenges.

What I tried to do for Mom was to gently enter her reality to calm her as best I could. It was an exhausting experience to find the right strategy that worked to soothe her and bring her back to herself. Usually, no amount of rational explanation worked, though I often found myself trying to explain things to Mom, an instinct I could not put aside. More often than not, I tried to improvise. Humor was often a fantastic tool, as was distraction. For example, I would drum my fingers on a nearby surface to the tune of the "William Tell Overture," and Mom would invariably start humming along. We'd get so riotous, we'd be singing at high volume and burst into laughter. That's how I fashioned my go-to rule: when in doubt, sing. Singing whatever came into my head often had the ability to distract Mom from her current mood or keep her engaged in the present.

Many of the ways in which Mom reacted or spoke could be understood in the context of Alzheimer's symptoms. For example, her random conversations originated from several different sources, and once we understood this, we could better appreciate the non-sequiturs and the reliance on past experiences that made her dialogue so bizarre.

Mom often incorporated words she heard around her into her conversation. If I told Daddy I found a letter in their mailbox, Mom would start talking about the man who lost his letter. Or she'd ask a question about someone who did something and put half of it away in the letter and the doctor outside (because one of us mentioned a doctor) gave her this ring (pointing to her ring) and what should she do?

I firmly believed Mom was trying to communicate with us. Part of this rambling was due to the fact that she couldn't recall the precise words she needed in order to explain herself. She talked around her subject, trying to create meaning with the words that did come to mind. I understand. When I speak my second, less extensive language (in this case Hebrew), I often substitute words to make myself understood. If I don't know how to say "divide," but I do know the word for "half," I can manage to say, "I'll take this half," instead of, "Let's divide this cake between us." (Yes, it's always about cake.)

She also talked about people or events in her past, often with great clarity. She could still recognize herself in childhood photos and even as a young twenty-year-old. Those past moments were accessible in her tangled brain whereas her present memories were all blank. It made sense that, if she was trying to understand the emotional map of her current surroundings, she pulled from her distant memory emotional experiences that were somehow similar. For example, when we giggled together, Mom would tell me I was her best friend and she knew me from school. In her mind, she was a young girl, the age where her strongest memories converged. It was too much to ask her to remember that she birthed me *just* fifty-three years ago.

Many of us experience delusions either when we are exhausted or pumped up on energy or drunk or when experiencing loss. We know what it was like to disconnect from reality, to believe something that isn't true. Thankfully, though, we come back to ourselves, as opposed to someone with Alzheimer's.

Despite not understanding the context of her present, Mom can and did experience a full range of emotions. The situation may not have been clear, but the emotions were. We didn't necessarily know what made her agitated or distressed, but these feelings flared in her as they flare in the rest of us. Sometimes she was happy; sometimes she was angry. She had an internal life that was every bit as vibrant as our own.

The challenge was to accept Mom in all her states. Loving, unpleasant, annoying, caring. Unable to hold significant, meaningful, coherent conversations. Unable to understand reality. But able to bond and feel and react in a nuanced world of her own making. Perception is in the eye of the beholder and I was ready to enter Mom's world to connect with her—to calm her when she was upset and to embrace her when she was content.

An article my brother Simon sent us from the *East Bay Times* in Concordia, California, that followed the disappearance of a woman with Alzheimer's and her eventual discovery, suggested that 60% of people with Alzheimer's wander at some time during the course of the disease because they are bored, overstimulated or confused.[8]

I understand why those three seemingly opposite states can produce the same results. And in fact, I feel that they are appropriate descriptions of Mom's experiences on a daily basis. When Mom was bored, she sat listlessly on the couch staring into space. If she shook herself out of that mood, it was often enough to induce her to start pacing or rummaging through the house.

---

[8] "Woman with Alzheimer's Wanders Away, Found," November 27, 2015, East Bay Times

Likewise, overstimulation, which went hand in hand with confusion, could cause her to dramatically rush from where she was to somewhere that she believed was safer—but if that was in the middle of town, she could endanger herself by dashing unthinkingly across the street. And then I was forced to follow, weaving my way through traffic to catch up to her.

On the positive side, Alzheimer's had made Mom into something of a poet.

"This mirror looks like me," she exclaimed once when we were walking by a wall of mirrors in the mall.

While not acknowledging her Alzheimer's per se, Mom was often aware that she couldn't remember as well as she used to.

"I don't know if I'm coming or going," she said, a phrase synonymous with her inability to gauge reality. "I don't know if I'm ready for what I'm waiting for."

Given what I knew about the toll this disease would take on my mom, it appeared that neither was I.

ოჯე

The kitchen is generally a place of pleasurable smells, defined tasks, and unhurried thinking. Of course, it helps that lemons and onions don't talk back or struggle against you when you need to use them. Like most vegetables, they are the perfect companions in times of stress.

God must have been playing a joke on us or perfecting his poetic imagery when the artichoke was created. It may be one of the most irrational foods there are. Its shapely leaves with individual thorns, and the strange "hair" that protects its heart create a fortress that we humans have had to ingeniously overcome in order to enjoy eating them. Perhaps it is delusional of us to think we can tame these strange thistles and make them edible. It doesn't stop us from trying, or taking the time to prepare them. Once they're cooked, they are a fun pleasure to eat. It's just that tiny end of the leaf that we grate against our teeth, that small taste of freshness that fills our mouths, before we toss the whole leaf away and it piles up with its brother and sister leaves to create a mountain of discarded plants. Then we make it to the heart, that larger surface of delectable flavor, something between asparagus and an eggplant that we must undress by removing its built-in shield before we can savor it. And all along, the sauce or dip that accompanies this dish has enhanced the flavor of the fruit to create a burst-in-your-mouth sensation. (Make sure you have plenty of sauce on hand in which to dip the leaves and *schmear* on the heart.) Eating an artichoke gives new meaning to the expression, "eat your heart out!"

Artichokes

I don't think I ever ate a fresh artichoke before coming to Israel. I learned the rudiments of preparation from a neighbor who was boiling up a pot of them with alluring lemon slices floating in the boiling water. It hooked me into making them for myself.

4-5 artichokes
Water
½ lemon, sliced
½ lemon, squeezed for juice

Sauce

Some people use melted butter as a sauce for the leaves. In our house, we like a simple mayo and mustard sauce, though there's also a garlicky sauce you can try.

Mayonnaise and Mustard Sauce
2 Tbsp mayonnaise
1 Tbsp mustard
Salt and pepper to taste

Mayonnaise and Garlic Sauce
2 Tbsp mayonnaise
1 Tbsp lemon juice
2-3 cloves garlic, crushed
Salt and pepper to taste

Directions:
Using a sharp pair of scissors, cut the artichoke stem then cut the point off each outer leaf. As leaves bunch closer together at the top, use a serrated knife to slice off the top of the artichoke. Soak each artichoke in water and white vinegar and clean by using your thumbs to bend and open

the inner-most part of the thistle to check for any stray bugs or snails (really, I have found snails in the middle of my artichoke). Place in a large pot with lemon slices and juice. Fill pot so water covers approximately two-thirds of the artichokes. Bring water to boil then keep on a low boil for one to two hours. Artichokes are ready to eat when the leaves remove easily with a small tug. To reveal the heart, once leaves are removed, use a spoon and gently scoop out the "choke." Discard choke and eat your heart out!

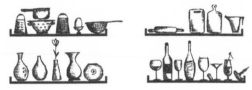

Immutable

Remember...and do not forget. (Deuteronomy 25:19)

The first time she reads
with alacrity
trying to gauge where he's gone
and when he'll return,
that blank space in her mind
shifting and unbalanced,
her mood like a plaintive love song.
She wants him home
where she can see him, tactile,
tethered to her the way the sun
once orbited the immutable earth.

"Why didn't he tell me?"
she asks the second time,
the countless repetitions
that led to his departure
are a story spun like cotton candy
sticking everywhere but her tangled brain.

Days pass.
As she remembers so she forgets,
again and again and again.
The folded paper,
the words,
his light-hearted tone:
her mouth curls in a tight scowl.

The morning after his return,
she wakes to see him next to her.
Wasn't he always here?

She finds the letter on the table and
reads as if for the first time.
"What is this?" she asks
setting it aside,
her sun restored to its orbit.

Chapter 8

Naomi in Wonderland

What do you do when your world literally turns upside down? In June 2016, Daddy called to tell me he'd been invited to attend a conference in Miami in September. As he was already going to the US, he decided he'd also travel to California to see my brother Simon. He was giving me advanced notice so that I could arrange to take the required holiday time from work. I had about three months to get used to the idea that I'd be with Mom on my own while Daddy was away for ten whole days.

As September drew near, I reminded myself that I'd done this before, albeit not for such a long period of time. I'd grown used to Mom's behavior. I also knew her schedule, and I would try to stick to it as much as possible. How bad could it get? The last time I'd taken care of Mom had been more than three years earlier, before we'd hired a caregiver. I knew I'd have good back up—Sahlee would be with us, and Rachel was a phone call away.

We threw logic out on day one, along with any concept of personal space and emotional buffers. The only time I was alone was when she was sleeping. I relied on my creative parenting skills and used her memory loss to keep her on schedule.

Once Mom was showered and dressed—a process I assisted her with—it was time to eat breakfast.

"Here are your medicines," I told her. "You have to put them in your mouth and swallow them with your juice."

"Those aren't mine," she stated.

"Can you put them in your mouth?"

"Why would I do that? I'm not taking those."

On the tenth try, she acquiesced. That was only because she couldn't remember I'd asked her to take them nine times previously!

She wanted to nap with her shoes and glasses on? Go ahead.

She wanted to eat her sandwich with a knife and fork? Great.

She wanted to do the dishes? Superb. Sahlee or I would wash them later with soap when she was sleeping.

She wanted to wear her clothes to bed? Fine with me.

When she asked where Daddy was, I told her he was at a conference (which was true) and that he'd be home soon (which was not so true). When she pouted that "he didn't tell me," I pulled out the note he'd left her:

Dear Naomi,
I have to go to a conference in Miami. I'll be back soon. Don't worry. Enjoy being with Miriam.
Love you very much,
Jack

That note was my most precious possession. I left it

lying on the kitchen table, but after that first day of Mom's constant questions, I decided I needed it with me at all times. It saved us from her anger at feeling abandoned.

Then it got really bad. Mom stood in the middle of her living room and told me in all earnestness that she needed to go home. I knew she had said similar things before, but now I was in charge. As the responsible adult, I had to use all my skills to help her find her way "home."

I tried telling her we were staying in the apartment just for the night. I used logic to show her the family photos, her name on their door, the familiar paintings. She told me she had a room identical to this one, but this one was not hers. She rebuffed my suggestions and angrily demanded I take her home. It was dark outside. Could I lock the door and walk to another room until she calmed down? Should I put music on and hope that that worked? Should we leave the apartment? What would happen if I took her outside? Would she run from me, or stubbornly refuse to return with me? I was terrified of her reaction, of losing all leverage to change the situation, of not being able to calm her.

I decided to chance it. We put our shoes on, gathered our purses, and set out into the night. We left from the front door of the apartment building and headed down the street, arm in arm, singing as we went. We turned the corner and continued walking round the block. We approached the building from the back entrance.

"Here's your building," I told her. "Here's your car. Let's go into the lobby. It's nice to be home. Let's go up the elevator to your apartment. Here's your door with your name on it. Here we are. We're home!"

She walked in appeased. And I trembled with relief.

"Thank you for bringing me home," she said as she put her purse under her pillow.

I told her we were having a girl's night, a slumber party.

"Can I get you anything?" Mom asked. "Do you need anything?"

How sweet her solicitousness was. I told her I was fine. Then she asked again and again and again until I exasperatedly told her that I could help myself.

Mom read Daddy's note one more time then finally climbed into bed and crashed till morning. While she was sleeping, I removed her purse, along with the skirt and shirt she had stuffed under her pillow, the extra nightie, the tissues and napkins she had collected, and her glasses that she'd folded with care.

My goal was to continue to find happiness together in each passing day. That was what I was aiming for. Our daily outings were, for the most part, serene. But nighttime brought its darkness with it.

None of the Alzheimer's books or websites prepared me for the rage Mom expressed. Or my helplessness and guilt when I couldn't defuse it.

I was stunned yet again by Mom's perception of reality. Comedian Steven Wright said it best: one morning he woke up and all his possessions had been replaced by exact copies.

Day six was the worst. We'd already walked out and come back twice. I'd even called her on the phone from the privacy of the study, pretending I was somewhere else to see if I could calm her.

She stood by the door for two hours. Two hours! She tried kicking it, using a nail file, even a wet rag. She gathered things for her journey—a book, her nightgown, four bras—and put on a winter coat. She appealed to my kindness to assist her in opening it, and when I wouldn't, cursed me and called me an imbecile and a schmuck (and worse things I won't mention). I kept telling her the door was locked until morning, that I'd take her home then but that we were staying here tonight. Nothing helped. Nothing I said seemed to make a dent in her determination to leave. She adamantly insisted that this was not her home and that she needed to go home to her parents.

I knew she was safe inside these walls. I had locked the top lock so she couldn't open the door even if she somehow succeeded in getting the right key in the regular lock. I had a momentary horrific image of her flinging open the large living room windows and jumping out in desperation from the third floor. Then I remembered with relief that the stiff blinds would block her from doing that.

So we rode it out, her periodic pleading, her anger. She was dripping with sweat in the humid living room. I tried my own mock anger to forestall hers. I tried rationalizing. I put on music. I busied myself so I wouldn't see her standing there. But I heard it, that intense turning of the door handle, the rattle of the keys being slid into and out of the lock, the mumbled words flung with fear to anyone who might be able to help. I wanted to cry seeing her standing there, feet planted by the door, her sloped back in the blue coat, sun hat askew on her head.

I don't know why she finally decided to listen. Perhaps she was just so worn out. I suggested we had to change our plans in light of the door being locked, that it was cool in her bedroom where the fan was on. I gently helped her take off the coat and wash her face in the bathroom. I led her to the bedroom and got her to sit with me. I fought my urge to suggest she undress and when she lay down fully clothed, I didn't care. She kept up a patter for another few minutes then drifted off to sleep.

I had had enough of the mercurial mood swings, of having no time to myself, of her thinking of Miriam as a little girl who was lost and needed to be found (all while she was holding my hand). I wanted no more of the loud cooing at every baby we saw, the same songs sung over and over and over and over, of feeling like her mother. I hated having to smile and talk at her level. I hated my bad moods and my monosyllabic sulk. I wanted to be in my own home with my husband and children and to sleep in my bed. I wanted my life back.

And yet…What would I have wished instead? What was the alternative? With all the pain and heartache we had, the future was only bleaker. So I would have to accept this mom, the one that stuffed my head with silly songs, who smiled and prattled on nonsensically, who laughed over corny jokes and was moved beyond words by a beautiful symphony. She was filled with love for her family, and particularly for me. When she asked how long she'd known me, I told her all my life, from the first kiss she gave me on the day that I was born. I knew this.

This was hard. This was so terribly hard. I'd lost my mom ten times over. But I could do this. I could treat her with the dignity she deserved as a sweet human being, as a beloved lost mother, as the competent woman who had birthed me. I vowed not to let her rage against the door again. I would walk out with her as many times as it took her to find her "home," and exhaust her in the process. For tomorrow, when she woke, there would be no memory of this incident. We would start again with the smiles and the songs. It would be my second chance (for the nth time…).

ഗ്രൗ

Mom was always such a giving person that she not only brought Daddy breakfast in bed every day throughout our childhood, but she made our school lunches and did the laundry until my brother Simon and I were both in high school. The downside of this generous behavior was that we were pampered children with few domestic skills. I even refused to do the laundry because the machines were in the eerie, creaky basement.

The one place where we always felt welcome, though, was the kitchen. Mom invited us to help her cook and we repeatedly witnessed the transformation of strange and often unappealing ingredients into delectable dishes. I still remember the slimy feel of trout even after it had been washed, the sight of bloody meat standing in the sink waiting for salting, and the joy of licking the bowl clean after the cake was in the oven.

Trouble started when we came back from college and vociferously voiced our objections to the traditional roles in our household, to the way Mom spoiled Daddy. Simon and I were products of the changing times in which we grew up, and our new intellectual environments fed our view of ourselves as enlightened. We wanted something different for ourselves, and ultimately succeeded in creating a more balanced life for our own families. My husband and brother both know how to cook and the women in our family hold degrees and maintain careers. In addition, we have made efforts to teach our own kids how to fend for themselves in the kitchen. They not only help out, they cook entire meals by themselves.

In the end, our objections didn't seem to make much impact on Mom and Daddy. Looking back, I realize that our role models weren't as poor as I judged them to be as a young adult. Domestic chores aside, the overall message I received was that I could be anything I wanted, learn and read whatever might be available, and follow the dreams that I aspired to. It was this education that empowered me to pursue my writing. I give the same message to my children—limitless doors to your future stand before you waiting to be opened.

In a loving, honest family like the one in which Simon and I grew up, our parents shouldered the responsibility of domestic labor so that we children could experience the world, as I find myself doing for my own children. Of course, I am thrilled that my husband shares equally in household chores and maintenance. But if a couple—like my parents—finds their balance with one partner taking on most of the cooking and cleaning, who am I to argue?

The fact that Shabbat rolls around every week means that I spend a lot of time in the kitchen preparing Shabbat meals. A friend once suggested that cooking for Shabbat was like cooking for Thanksgiving on a weekly basis. Sometimes it's downright tiring to exert that much energy. I rely on my cooking experience to create a balanced menu. I am always open to trying new recipes. When my husband Jeff and I visit our siblings, the fun of being together is always enhanced by the good food they make. Here are some of the recipes we've shared along the way to establishing our own home.

Onion Quiche

I started making quiche when I was in Oberlin College, saving money by cooking and eating at a vegetarian food cooperative. It is a recipe I know by heart and it takes me about twenty minutes to get this quiche in the oven. I've made it for family gatherings and special events in our community. It is a standard and well-loved dish in our house. When my kids were young, they voted this their favorite dish over pizza and hamburgers. If you have kids who don't like onions, place them on only half the quiche. Or, use alternative vegetables like mushrooms or sautéed squash.

Crust:
1½ cups flour
½ cup canola oil
5 Tbsp cold water
1 tsp salt

Filling:
1 large onion, sliced in rings
1 Tbsp canola oil for frying
1½ cups grated yellow cheese (Cheddar or American)

Custard:
4 eggs
1½ cups milk
¼ tsp salt
1 tsp prepared mustard
1 Tbsp flour
Paprika

Directions:

Sauté onions until translucent. Let cool. In a bowl, mix crust ingredients and pat into round nine-inch / twenty-three-cm pie pan. Using the same bowl, mix custard ingredients, making sure to smooth any lumps. In pie pan, place layer of grated cheese at bottom of crust, then onions on top. Pour custard on top and gently push down with a fork any onions sticking up. Sprinkle top with paprika. Bake for forty-five minutes at 350 degrees F / 180 degrees C.

Lettuce Wraps with Ground Beef

My sister-in-law Sharon in California taught me how to make these. With her spacious kitchen and fun cooking gadgets, I especially enjoyed chopping the peanuts. These wraps have become one of our mainstays.

1 lb / ½ kilo ground beef
2 garlic cloves, crushed
1 carrot, grated
½ cup cabbage, grated
¼ cup chopped peanuts (can use walnuts)
3 spring onions, chopped
Salt and pepper to taste
1 cup soy ginger dressing (or equivalent sauce)
10 washed lettuce leaves

Directions:
Sauté garlic in a big pot. Add meat, draining the liquid when meat is cooked. Add carrots, cabbage and peanuts and simmer for twenty minutes. Pour on soy ginger sauce and add spring onions and mix well. Remove from heat. Place a small amount of filling on a lettuce leaf, turn up the bottom and sides, and wrap as if wrapping a tortilla.

Mexican-Style Chicken

I first tasted this dish at my other sister-in-law Sharon's home in New Jersey. It is a hearty and filling way to cook chicken in winter, with just enough piquant to startle the taste buds.

8-10 chicken pieces
1 Tbsp olive oil
1 onion, sliced in strips
3 cloves garlic, crushed
3 peppers of various colors, sliced in strips
2 tsp cumin
2 tsp salt
Pepper to taste
1 12-oz / 340 gr can black beans or baked beans
1 16-oz / 580 gr can spicy kidney beans

Directions:
Sauté garlic and onions in oil until translucent. Add multi-colored peppers and spices and cook another ten minutes. In a bowl, mix beans and add cooled peppers. Place chicken pieces in large oven dish and pour beans on top. Bake covered for one hour at 350 degrees F / 180 degrees C. Uncover and bake another ten minutes.

Uncle Ze'ev's Brownies

Sometimes I purposely undercook this dessert to make the brownies melt in your mouth. Even though I've been making this recipe for years, my brother-in-law Ze'ev still makes the best brownies around.

1 cup flour
1 cup cocoa
1 tsp baking powder
1 tsp salt
2 cups sugar
4 eggs
2 tsp vanilla
¾ cup canola oil
½ cup chocolate chips (optional)

Directions:
Mix dry ingredients. Add eggs, vanilla and oil and mix well. Pour into eight-inch / twenty-cm pan. For an extra chocolaty taste, add chocolate chips. Bake at 350 degrees F / 180 degrees C for approximately thirty minutes.

Lemons

Eight lemons fill the sink
plucked this morning from my tree
which we planted when we first arrived.

I wash them,
roll them on the counter
to make them pliant.
A scented mist erupts from their peel.
From one, I cut a small wedge
to reveal delicate flesh
as we are commanded
because the Land is holy.

We squeeze the lemons,
drink our fill of tart juice,
grate the rind for zest,
suck on the empty halves still laden
with pulp, take what we love,
carry within us this one tree,
not only the fruit but its planting,
not only its growth but its roots.

There are days we live this dream
as if death will not find us, the joy
of ripe lemons, fragrant fingers,
a leafy tree with white blossoms,
of having enough.

after Li-Young Lee

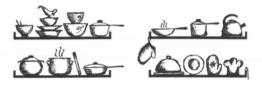

Chapter 9

The Nakedness of my Mother

There was a verse in Leviticus that unwittingly caught my attention: "The nakedness of your father and the nakedness of your mother you shall not uncover. She is your mother; you must not uncover her nakedness (18:7)."

Instinctively, I knew that this prohibition and the following biblical prohibitions were related to sexual transgressions. But the unwanted intimacies I have shared with Mom made me feel as if I was transgressing in a different way.

When I was about ten or eleven, Simon and I often played hide-and-seek in our house. Once, I was under the dresser in my parent's room holding back a sneeze from all the dust when I heard footsteps along the hall heading straight towards me. I peered out from my hiding place to see if Simon was close, my vision truncated by the bottom of the dresser. Instead of short little legs, I saw my father's shoed feet and brown pants. He must have been going out that night because as I watched, he took off his

119

shoes and then his pants. All of a sudden, I felt squeamish about being in that spot. What would happen if Daddy completely undressed and I saw him naked? Should I call out to tell him where I was? Would he be angry with me? Would I be in more trouble if I stayed silent?

I couldn't see much—which wasn't quite the point—but I was conscious of violating some iron-clad rule that I must not invade my parent's privacy. In a voice quaking with fear, I called out to Daddy. He bent down to see where I was then quickly pulled on some pants. Thankfully, he was more amused than anything as he showed me out and shut the door behind me.

I haven't been so lucky with avoiding Mom's private moments. The nature of Alzheimer's means that Mom has trouble remembering the sequence of things and how to do them, what comes first and why there's an order. She can become angry in the mornings, perhaps overwhelmed by the number of tasks associated with preparing ourselves for the day. And she won't ask for help. Alzheimer's has robbed her of that ability.

Whenever I stayed over to be with Mom, it was my job to assist with her hygiene in the mornings. When Mom awoke, she automatically entered the bathroom and prepared for a shower. I used the excuse that I, too, needed to shower, and Mom reluctantly allowed me into the bathroom. It was a heavy burden to see Mom—confused, fragile—as she ineffectively prepared to take a shower. Mom tolerated my presence there because she trusted me, yet this very trust put us in conflict. I was privy to her most intimate moments, something I had been taught as a child was unacceptable. Somehow it felt like a betrayal of Mom.

Standing in the bathroom, Mom would take off her nightgown but forget to remove her underpants. The water had to be turned on and set to the right temperature.

Then it was time to actually step into the water and wash with soap. I had to persuade her to take off her remaining clothes and enter the shower. She absolutely refused to wash her hair. For some reason, that feeling of warm water enveloping her as she stood under the shower frightened Mom. Her showers lasted under one minute. She often forgot to wash off the soap.

To see myself reflected in Mom's overweight, aging body was unnerving. I secretly prayed that I would not end up as she had. I reminded myself that when she was younger, Mom had cared about her appearance. It was only the last couple of years as her Alzheimer's became more pronounced that she had stopped caring. It gave me comfort to think that my own daughter might not only learn from my patient example of honoring my mother, but would also step in to help me if I ever needed it.

Once we were through with the shower, and I had helped Mom wipe herself with her towel, we entered her bedroom to get her dressed. Mom was incapable of choosing her own clothes, and for the most part, the clothing items confused her. Sometimes she was open to our assisting her, and sometimes she thought we were making her out to be incompetent. Why, she wondered, should we involve ourselves in her private matters? Her anger flared in these moments, anger expressed in an increasingly halting manner as she searched for words that just wouldn't come.

As part of our effort to streamline the dressing process, we made sure that Mom's skirts had elastic waists and that shirts and sweaters had as few buttons as possible. Her shoes closed with Velcro and opened wide enough to slip on effortlessly.

Mom's undergarments were the real success story. We had effectively shopped to find large, attractive cotton underpants with snug—but not tight—elasticated waist and leg openings, and, best of all, bras that were soft, relaxed, front-closing and comfortable.

The most difficult item of apparel that Mom had to negotiate daily was her bra. First she had to twist herself into knots to hook the bra around her waist, then slide it backward, hiking it up to the right position to finally stick her arms, elbow-first, through the thin straps and fit her breasts into the cups that were meant to be supportive.

When we entertained the idea of finding bras that were easier to put on, I did have thoughts that Mom should go bra-less, but if she was still going out in public, she really needed something to support her.

When I started to investigate bra options, I discovered that there were quite a few alternatives to the standard bras: bras that closed in the front with zippers, snaps, large hooks-and-eyes, even ties. There were shirts that tightly hugged the chest, sports bras that were soft and provided support much like a halter top. There was even something called the BreastNest, a type of tank-top support for large breasted women. I was optimistic enough to believe that many of these bras were designed not only to make money but to bring comfort to women, many with dementia or with arthritis who lose dexterity in their fingers.

The close-in-the-front bras also assist caregivers in helping dress their charges. We found and ordered our bras on line by searching, "front closing bras for elderly."

There were frustrating times when I wanted to hurry Mom along in her dressing, but I was reminded again of a quote from the *AlzLive* digital newspaper: "It is important to enable a person with dementia to make their own choices for as long as they can and, if they do need assistance, to offer it tactfully and sensitively…If the person is determined to wear a hat in bed or a heavy coat in summer, try to respect their choice, unless it might cause harm."[9] Words to live by.

❦❦❦

I tried to avoid situations where I was responsible for Mom's hygiene, not because I didn't want to take care of her but because it meant again putting myself in her intimate space.

The problem with this attitude was that I often noticed too late that Mom's body needed attention.

Once, I noticed too late that Mom needed to reach the bathroom. Before I could help her get there, she had wet not only herself but the couch on which she was sitting. Mom was far from incontinent, but she did often become puzzled as to what to do in the bathroom. Sometimes, she even forgot where the bathroom was. I could envision a time when we would have to buy adult pull-ups for her to wear instead of underpants, which would cover any small accidents she had. Diapering her in adult diapers, though, something that was bound to happen in the future, was beyond my current comprehension.

I thought it would be easy to entice Mom to get her fingernails cut. When I first became aware of needing to cut them, I could see how long they'd gotten, and how many had cracked as if they were thin pieces of paper.

"I don't need anyone to cut my nails," Mom stated as I tried to get her to sit still for me. "I'll do them later."

I knew she couldn't do them later, so I persisted, making a game of it and inviting her to Chez Cohen Nail Salon.

---

[9] "Tips for Helping a Person with Dementia to Dress," Alzlive.com, Team AlzLive

"Where is it?" she asked.

"Right here in your living room," I replied.

The novelty worked, and she did let me cut them. These days, I cut them regularly by putting her in front of the TV with a movie on so that she is distracted. And while she watches and sings along to her favorite scenes, I snip with abandon.

Feet and toenails were an altogether different matter. Even though Mom showered almost every day, she did not clean or wipe between her toes. It was only by chance one summer morning before Mom put on her knee highs and sandals, that I realized that Mom had a serious fungus problem.

Yes, I had cleaned my children's urine, their bowel movements, their vomit, but somehow having to deal with Mom's stinky feet was almost too much. I decided to take her for a pedicure so that someone else would do the work of cutting the nails and cleaning her feet.

When the pedicurist took off Mom's shoes, one of her nails was completely bloody and there was blood between her toes and on her knee high stocking. We were both shocked to see it. We quickly discovered that one nail had grown so ragged it had pierced the skin on the toe next to it. The blood had congealed under the nail, turning it temporarily black.

It was pointless asking Mom if her toes had been hurting her. They must have been. I wondered how she could have walked through the obvious pain.

As I bent to see her toes, I noticed a big bruise on Mom's knee. Daddy had told me she'd fallen the previous week and was still complaining of pain in her side. Here was another sign of her fall.

We did not intentionally overlook Mom's health issues. We just forgot that Mom needed us more than she was able to express. The hard part was not only forcefully intruding on her privacy but also getting her to allow us to help her. Thankfully, Mom only grumbled a little during the pedicure. We kept her busy singing songs. Before we left the salon, we made a follow-up appointment for the coming month.

The pedicurist had been hesitant to commit to another appointment. When the time rolled around for the next visit, I called ahead to make sure she was still willing to take Mom on as a client. I also asked if there was an available slot with "Pierre," the French hairdresser who had been cutting Mom's hair for about twenty years. Mid-week, before the double appointment, the pedicurist called to say that she was unwilling to cut Mom's nails. She did not want to be liable in case Mom made any sudden movements that caused her harm. Reluctantly I told her I understood but that we'd be there for the hair appointment.

Pierre was also hesitant. He'd seen Mom become more confused and unpredictable due to her Alzheimer's. I assured him that I'd be there too, and that Mom doted on him, often giving him glorious greetings when she saw him in the street outside his salon.

We showed up early for the appointment, the August heat and humidity having left its toll on us as we wandered in the city. Pierre turned as we entered then returned to the client in his chair. I apologized that we were early.

The small salon was crowded. As I went to move some chairs for Mom to sit down, I heard Pierre speak.

"I can't," he said, his back to us.

"What?" I asked.

"I can't."

"What do you mean you can't? You can't what, cut her hair?"

"I can't."

"But I spoke to you last week. We made an appointment with you."

Not once did Pierre come over to greet us or try to speak to us in private. Neither did he turn around and face us.

I could not believe that Pierre had so openly rejected us. Oh, I boiled up and over. Unfortunately, my anger made me tongue-tied. I yelled out some indistinct adjectives and stormed off in a huff, Mom and our caregiver Sahlee following behind. Except I couldn't really storm off, not like I wanted to. Mom's gait was so slow I had to significantly reduce my walking speed to match hers.

Even as I fumed, Sahlee pointed out several other salons in the street where we were walking. "He's not the only hairdresser," she said.

Hey, I thought, *you're right!*

We stopped at one of the salons, and I entered cautiously. I engaged the hairdresser in a short discussion, explaining that Mom had Alzheimer's but that it shouldn't hinder him while cutting her hair. Yossi was nonplussed. He said hello to Mom, invited his assistant to wash her hair, then expertly began cutting and shaping Mom's silver locks.

Let me describe our new hero: shoulder-length black hair with streaks of Bordeaux, nut-brown skin, deep eye crinkles, a trim mustache, tight black pants and T-shirt, and these tri-colored shoes in dayglow yellow, pink, and green. Did I mention handsome? Mom was in heaven. She praised the hands of the assistant who had washed her hair then chatted amiably with Yossi about London, one of Yossi's favorite cities and Mom's birth place.

When we left, we were all in good moods. Mom certainly had no recollection of what had transpired, but I purposely led us home in a circuitous route so that we would not have to pass Pierre's salon.

That was the first time I had faced outright prejudice toward Alzheimer's. I understood Pierre's professional dilemma. What I didn't understand was how he had treated a respected client. With a restored faith in humanity due to Yossi's openness, I reclaimed my ability to express myself. Here's what I wanted to say to Pierre.

"Pierre, you lost our business today. Instead of treating Mom with kindness, you ostracized her because you view her as sick. You had the audacity to embarrass us in a roomful of strangers by literally turning your back on us. Your lack of empathy dehumanized Mom. Had you made the effort to find the best and safest way to cut Mom's hair, you would have been rewarded with the emotional warmth she bestows on those around her. If this is the way you treat valued customers, we are happy to move on."

There. Enough said. It took time, but we even found a new pedicurist.

ↄ◞◠ↄ

Mom's fingers were also in danger of being overlooked. Mom's rings were tight on her fingers. I kept noticing them, saying we had to do something about getting the rings off her fingers, then not acting on it.

How often do we take the time to notice—really notice—the state of someone's physical condition in an intimate way? Who really wants to wash and dress their parent, cut their nails or assist them in using the toilet?

Mom had not removed the rings in many years and her fingers had shaped themselves around them, growing and fattening until the rings were unable to slide off or even wiggle. We tried removing them with soap, even oil, but they would not budge. I realized we needed professional assistance.

Mom had been wearing the same five rings as long as I can remember. The first was her engagement ring. The original diamond had been bought from a store owned by Daddy's Uncle Abe in London. It was a flawed diamond, which they only found out after purchase. Many years later, my grandmother's neighbor passed on a diamond to Mom after her death; Mom had the new diamond reset in her engagement ring. The second was her platinum wedding band, patterned and wide, which would prove the hardest to remove because platinum is harder than gold and silver. The third was a big jade stone on a gold band that Daddy had brought back with him from a trip to Hong Kong. The fourth was a silver ring made by Yemenite jewelers who lived in Ekron, just outside of Rehovot, purchased in 1976, the year my family spent in that city. And the fifth was a wide silver ring from Rhodes, Greece, with a traditional Greek key pattern.

I knew not to attempt to have the rings removed without my dad present. Mom defers to Daddy in all things, even bringing him her empty plate after lunch so that he can confirm that, yes, she should place it in the sink. If I suggest something like, "Here, Mom, you can put your plate in the sink," she'll ask Daddy for his approval. In her eyes, he is the sun and the moon and the stars, all-knowing and benevolent.

We had spoken to Mom several times about removing her rings. She would always acquiesce and say, "Yes, of course, I'll come with you to the jewelers." In the first store we entered, when she realized what we were up to, Mom became hostile. I quietly told the silversmith that Mom had Alzheimer's but she heard me and called me all manner of foul names for suggesting she was ill. Rather than coerce her, we left the store and did other chores.

As we walked on the high street of Netanya, I suggested to Daddy that we visit a specific jewelry store where we had been previously and where the proprietor was friendly. I told him that I would enter the store first and see if Eva, the owner, could help us.

When I described the situation and pointed to my parents standing outside the store, she was kind enough to agree to help. She won Mom's confidence with her gentle manner and friendly voice.

She walked us up a small alley to where her silversmith worked then stroked Mom's palms while the silversmith got his pliers and cut across the shank of each ring. Both Eva and the silversmith tut-tutted at the state of Mom's tight rings and told us it was good that we'd come.

And then it was done. And I felt joyous. We'd brought Mom through this difficult procedure intact and without incident. Her fingers have large white patches on them where the rings were previously, but their shape is already changing, her fingers breathing and spreading out instead of being confined by the tight rings. We'll get the rings resized, but for the moment, Mom doesn't even remember she once wore rings. Her fingers had been laid bare and I—briefly and humbly—averted my gaze.

❧❧

As a young girl, I was conscious of Mom being a social creature, one who made friends easily and who bestowed kindnesses on her friends. It is this aspect of her personality that shines when she interacts with friends, patient shop owners or even complete strangers. She was also a giving, loving mother, especially when I was going through my awkward and rebellious teenage years. That loving nature has been amplified by her Alzheimer's.

Each week when I arrived, Mom's greetings were always effusive. "I haven't seen you in so long," she'd say, pulling me to her in a tight hug. I wanted to tell her that I was here last week and the week before but it didn't really matter.

"When was the last time I saw you?" she'd ask. "It's been ages."

After I was showered with kisses, more hugs and more kisses, we got down to business. We would sit in the living room enjoying each other's company and the rich sunshine bathing the room in bright strips. Mom wandered off to make tea, asking several times how to make it and what I wanted in it. My preference was always for herbal tea, but if she brought me something different that was okay too.

I noticed that Mom was relaxed and—dare I say it— happy. She smiled and chatted easily. She had not yet burned the plastic electric kettle by placing it on the gas stove or dropped the glass jar of spaghetti sauce on the floor or lost her glasses for the hundredth time or forgotten that we had had tea together just 20 minutes earlier. Perhaps it was her new medicine, Ebixa (memantine).[10] It was specifically meant to calm her and it seemed to be working.

We made plans to meet Daddy for lunch at a new sushi place in town. Mom claimed she remembered the restaurant. She was sure we had eaten there only days ago, and that we'd been there many times.

Working body, wandering mind. Was that better than keeping your mind and losing your body? I asked my friend Evelyn who, in her nineties, was slowing down

---

[10] Memantine is a drug that treats moderate to severe Alzheimer's. It can improve or stabilize the cognitive (thinking, learning and memory) and daily functioning of Alzheimer's patients.

considerably. Bouts of sciatica, loss of vision, and aching joints accompanied her wherever she went. Evelyn was all there mentally, played complicated word games most weekends, and could even remember the names of all of her forty-five-plus precious great-grandchildren.

"There is no good answer to that question. You take the cards you are dealt," Evelyn reflected in her no-nonsense manner.

There was comfort in realizing that when Mom did get worse, she wouldn't remember her aches and pains. She'd be immune to the changes occurring in her body, protected by her mind.

e/ɔe/ɔ

Mom isn't the only one with memory problems. There are two recipes that I requested from Mom more than once because wherever I placed the first written copy was a mystery to me. So I'd call her and ask again. I finally got smart and stashed them in a place where I knew I could locate them in a pinch.

Saigon Chicken

I keep this recipe in the middle of a cookbook so I know where to find it, though the paper is stained and torn. Mom had given me this recipe many years ago written out in her own hand. I lost that copy and then requested it again. When I take out the recipe, it reminds me of her fragility.

2 chickens, cut into 8 pieces
1½ tsp curry powder
1½ tsp granulated garlic or 2 cloves fresh
½ cup honey
1 30 oz / 850 gr can crushed pineapples with juice
1 cup flour for dredging

Directions:
Coat each chicken piece in a thin layer of flour by dredging it in a small bowl of flour. Place in baking pan. In separate bowl, mix pineapple and other ingredients, including juice from the pineapple. Pour over chicken and bake covered at 350 degrees F / 180 degrees C for one hour. Uncover and bake another fifteen minutes until browned.

Sweet and Sour Squash

Mom gave this recipe to me early in my married life. I've lost it several times over the years, only to call and ask for it again. I copied it into my recipe collection, a small three-ring binder that Mom gave me once as a present. Not too long ago, when I was preparing a dinner for guests after my son Rafi's wedding, I asked Mom to slice the squash as a help to me and as a way to keep her involved in the busy proceedings. I had only turned away for a minute before I realized she had grated the squash by hand. We made a squash kugel instead.

4-5 large squash, sliced into circles
1 large onion, chopped
1 28 oz / 800 gr can crushed tomatoes
2 Tbsp tomato paste
Juice of 1 lemon (3 Tbsp)
¼ cup brown sugar
Salt and pepper to taste

Directions:
In a large pot, sauté onions. When onions are translucent, add squash and sauté for five min. Combine tomato, sugar and lemon. Pour over squash and bring to boil. Simmer for twenty minutes.

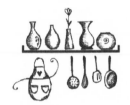

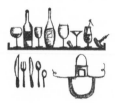

Two Toothbrushes

She sang that crazy song
when I was five:
two toothbrushes fall in love,
marry in haste, share the same toothpaste.
How I'd brush and brush
just to keep her singing.
I am the blue toothbrush and she, the pink.
She is such a sweet toothbrush.
We've met somewhere before,
by the bathroom door
of my memory,
my elbow jutting gently into her side
with each brushing motion,
and once I was the pink toothbrush
glowing from her attentions,
my nylons bristling and whistling.

I tell myself this song keeps her healthy.

Or maybe I'm singing to relive that moment
when I was still her child.

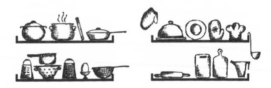

Chapter 10

Charms to Soothe a Savage Breast

A chance visit by a friend and her two-year-old had me digging out the baby toys in our storage cupboard. We raced cars, played with a tool set, and shook all the noise-makers in the house. The rattles were such fun, especially the rain rattle, whose brightly-colored plastic beads cascaded through a series of levels to create the sound of rain.

If I as a fairly competent adult could enjoy this toy, maybe Mom would too. She loved music so much that it might be an alternative way to reach her, as she had become more child-like in her interactions with people, including myself.

I put aside a small tambourine, a drum, bells, and the rain rattle, and took them with me on my next visit. Mom and I started by making random sounds then played an "echo" game where she would repeat the simple rhythm I created. We worked our way into "Raindrops Keep Falling on my Head," "April Showers," and "Singing in the Rain."

We were having such fun, I almost forgot that I was "playing" with Mom as I had once played with my children. All of a sudden, I became uncomfortable with my role. Who, I asked myself, was the child here? I didn't like the idea of being Mom's mother. But circumstances had pushed us to this relationship. I took a deep breath and let it go. The broad smile on Mom's face was all that I needed to realize I'd hit upon a positive activity.

In fact, whatever else was going on in Mom's brain, music had remained a constant source of comfort for her. Mom had attended a weekly classical music concert almost since her arrival in Israel twenty years ago. Hosted by She'arim Netanya, the "Music at Midday" concerts showcased talented immigrant musicians for a one-hour program—be it piano and other soloists, opera singers, or quartets—with the funds collected going directly to the musicians.

Mom had once volunteered to publicize the concerts in the local papers. She would sit on the phone for hours with the director of the program to write out the various weekly concert schedules. Then she'd type it up and send it by email to the addresses she'd collected. The earlier in the week she accomplished this task, the better, as the papers needed advanced time to print the information. Mom became easily flustered when deadlines were rushed because the director couldn't give her what she needed in time. When it was clear that Mom could no longer handle the pressures of the job, the director of the program gave Mom a new task, one befitting her decreased capabilities: Mom would come to the hall early to arrange chairs. Chair-arranging was something Mom could handle. It kept her feeling a part of the concerts themselves for a good few years. For the past three years, though, Mom has just shown up for the musical experience.

Some members of the audience had been coming to the concerts as long as Mom had, and over the years, through my own attendance, I'd met many of them. There were at least two other individuals with Alzheimer's who attend on a regular basis. They'd sit in the same seats almost every week, often showing up early to drink tea together. One man sat quietly in the corner, often stroking a stuffed animal. He'd tap his cane along to the music, to the annoyance of the other listeners, until his caregiver gently took it away. Sadly, he passed away in 2018. The other individual was constantly clowning, especially with Mom.

The strange banter and crazy word jokes that would go on between them was hilarious. Except that if you'd heard it once, you'd hear it again each time they were together. The good news was that he didn't remember he'd told these jokes before, and Mom reacted as if they were new each time she heard them.

Once the music started, Mom's attention was steadfast. She was infused with joy, often humming along or even clapping to more mainstream pieces. The concerts had become weekly music therapy for her.

In his book *Musicophilia: Tales of Music and the Brain,*[11] Oliver Sacks examines ways in which music "talks" to people with different neurological diseases. When it comes to Alzheimer's, he suggests that music therapy connects with the passions, cognitive powers, memories and thoughts of the individual to stimulate them, enrich and enlarge their existence, and to give them a sense of constancy, freedom and centeredness.[12]

It didn't matter if Mom couldn't remember who I

---

[11] Sacks, Oliver, *Musicophilia: Tales of Music and the Brain*, Vintage Books, New York, 2007
[12] Ibid, pp 372-373

was or where she was or even how she got dressed that morning. The music somehow allowed her to find her "self" again, that inner core of her desires and emotions that made her unique. It brought to the fore those personality traits that seemed to exist despite the failing cognitive functions that Mom experienced.

Having read Sacks' book, I learned about a documentary called *Alive Inside.*[13] Watching the movie was a redemptive experience. It spoke directly to me in its message that music makes a difference to someone with Alzheimer's at almost every stage of the disease.

The film follows Dan Cohen, executive director of Music and Memory,[14] who in 2006, volunteered to create individual musical play lists for residents of a nursing home in New York. Most of the individuals he worked with were in late stages of Alzheimer's; many sat all day in a comatose-like state. Cohen discovered that when they listened to music that was specifically tailored to their taste, history and background, they literally and shockingly came to life, becoming more coherent and interactive, often for the first time in years.

Cohen's program of introducing music into the lives of nursing home patients was so profound in its results that it has now been copied in hundreds of facilities in the US and Canada.

Music in films, especially musicals from her youth, appeal to Mom's musical memory. Once, when Mom's sister Barbara was visiting, they started singing songs from a 1954 film, *Carmen Jones,* an adaptation of Bizet's *Carmen* with an all-African American cast. Mom hadn't

---

[13] *Alive Inside: A Story of Music and Memory,* Michael Rossato-Bennett, Projector Media, January 18, 2014.

[14] Music and Memory is the organization founded by Dan Cohen to bring music to dementia patients. Their website is musicandmemory.org.

seen the movie in more than thirty years, but she remembered the lyrics and complicated syncopation to the music.

When I tire of watching shows like *Annie Get Your Gun, Easter Parade*, or *Singing in the Rain,* I play a movie that has enchanted millions of young children since it came out in 2013, Disney's *Frozen.*[15]

When we watch *Frozen*, Mom is charmed by the opening voices and graceful snowflakes. She laughs when she sees the trolls, and she comments many times about the cold and snow. As we watch Elsa and Anna struggle to assert their sisterly love, it moves me to think of the sacrifices we make for the people we love dearly. What Disney movies have is a clear and explicit visual language that is easily interpreted. Add in colorful scenes, catchy songs, and unambiguous emotions, and it was easy to see why Mom enjoys this animated movie.

Alzheimer's patients can also be "awakened" through drawing, painting and other crafts where they take up familiar hands-on projects. I've heard about one man whose family discovered that he loved to fill in forms. It didn't matter what he wrote on the applications he would complete; what mattered was the stimulation he received from signing his name and randomly filling in responses.

I relied on music every time I visited with Mom. We sang and danced in the living room, as we walked down the stairwell in their apartment, on the streets of the city, or as an activity in the afternoons. We watched old musicals like *An American in Paris, West Side Story* and *Oklahoma.* We sang folk songs and ballads from *Rise Up*

---

[15] *Frozen*, Jennifer Lee and Chris Buck, Disney, November 28, 2013.

Singing,[16] which included old British favorites like "Cockles and Muscles," and "With Her Head Tucked Underneath Her Arm," a humorously dark song about the ghost of Anne Boleyn. And often, when she climbed into bed at the end of the day, sometimes as early as seven p.m., Daddy would put on music in her bedroom where she conducted symphonies or listened to vintage Beatles.

On one recent afternoon, I used it to dispel Mom's depression.

"Everything is weird. I feel like a weird person," Mom said when she woke up from her nap. "My brain's not functioning."

Mom had said those kinds of things before. This time, I was determined to distract her, but even as we drank tea together, Mom continued to tell me about her fears.

"I had horrible dreams about you," she said. "I didn't know who was in charge. It's happening, one weird thing after another."

I tried again to steer the conversation to other things, and again Mom circled back to the same negative feelings. "Everything is upside down inside me. I don't know what I'm doing. I feel very strange at the moment. I feel depressed. All the things I'm supposed to do but haven't done. I don't think I'm up to scale."

I knew that talk alone would not banish Mom's mood as she would not remember what we had said to each other. So I got out the musical instruments. We banged out tunes from *Carmen* with our castanets and tambourines. We pulled up music on her USB and sang along with Barbara Streisand's lyrical voice. We danced to the music of Michael Bolton. Then we sat down on the

---

[16] Patterson, Annie and Peter Blood, ed., *Rise Up Singing,* Sing Out, USA and Canada, 1988.

couch and took some selfies, giggling all the while. When we reviewed the photos, Mom pointed to herself and said, "She has a nice smile." (And she did.)

Music restored Mom's sense of joy. I saw it every time we were together. When we sang, Mom's memory was active, and she derived so much pleasure from it.

Much of the music we listened to and movies we watched had been lovingly provided to us by my brother Simon. Simon did not live in close proximity to my parents. Despite his distance from us, he was firmly on this journey with my father and me, seeing things from his own unique perspective and making us laugh with his boisterous humor.

❧❀❧

I could not necessarily imagine what was going on in Mom's brain, but when I was working in the kitchen and listening to music, I, too, could enter a state where I was focused on my tasks in calm and contentment.

There are several foods that remind me of brains. Broccoli is more like "baby trees," the description Mom used on me when I was little to get me to eat it (and peas, of course, were "baby balls"). But cauliflower and cabbage, well, they definitely remind me of the human brain.

When I'm cutting and soaking cauliflower, I marvel at the beautiful florets with their hiding places for green and white bugs or black bugs smaller than a pin head. I carefully clean them, knowing they hold secrets I may never recognize.

Sometimes cutting white cabbage suggests slicing into a brain. It's the closest I'll ever come, though my brother-in-law Ze'ev has experimented on rat brains as part of his research as professor of anatomy and neuroscience at Ben-Gurion University of the Negev. I imagine

143

that a cabbage is more like a healthy brain than a diseased Alzheimer's brain is. We are big salad eaters. We have several favorite cabbage salads, all fresh and crisp.

Roasted Cauliflower with Tehina

This eye-catching dish is a great way to prepare cauli-flower. The combination of tehina and date honey adds a burst of flavor to every bite. Enjoy!

1 large head cauliflower
2 Tbsp olive oil
Salt to taste
2 Tbsp tehina
1-2 Tbsp date honey
¼ cup chopped parsley
Pomegranate seeds

Directions:
Cut cauliflower into large florets. Toss with oil and salt and place on a large baking sheet for twenty-five minutes at 420 degrees F / 210 degrees C. Remove to cool in a serving dish. Drizzle with tehina and honey. Garnish with pomegranates and parsley. Serve warm.

Cabbage Salad: Four Variations

The following four dressings can be added to half a head of a large cabbage thinly sliced with a sharp knife. Cutting it with a knife instead of putting it through a shredder makes a thicker, tactile salad. Or try using a large hand-held peeler for thinner slices.

Oil and Vinegar

¾ cup vegetable oil
¼ cup white vinegar (may substitute apple cider vinegar)
1 clove garlic, crushed
1 tsp salt (or to taste)
1 tsp dried basil
½ tsp dried oregano
3 Tbsp lemon juice
¼ cup fresh parsley, chopped
Pepper to taste

Mustard and Rice Vinegar

3 cloves garlic, crushed
2 Tbsp lemon juice
2 Tbsp rice vinegar
½ tsp prepared Dijon mustard
1 pinch red pepper flakes
⅓ cup canola oil
Salt and pepper to taste
¼ cup sunflower seeds

Lemon and Date Honey[17]

¼ cup lemon juice (preferably freshly squeezed)
2 Tbsp vegetable oil
2 Tbsp white vinegar
2Tbsp date honey
Salt to taste
¼ cup toasted almonds, slivered
¼ cup fresh parsley, chopped
½ cup craisins

Mayonnaise and Mustard

½ cup mayonnaise
¼ cup whole grain mustard
2 Tbsp lemon juice
2 Tbsp sugar
Salt and pepper to taste

Directions:
Slice the cabbage thinly using a large sharp knife and place in a large bowl. In a closed container, mix dressing ingredients. Combine cabbage and dressing, and add remaining ingredients if any. Marinate for up to two hours before serving.

---

[17] Based on "Cabbage and Cranberry Salad," *Cook in Israel: Home Cooking Inspiration*, Orly Ziv, 2013.

Promises

If you had asked if I was happy
that summer the peaches shriveled
on the tree and we roamed the malls
buying our desires like so much forbidden fruit;
if you had asked as I settled in the house,
the kids returning to eat and leave
their dirty laundry and
you washed the darks in hot water
and *pinked* my new shirt;
when I knocked wine on the floor
and glass cut my leg,
or even as we marked another anniversary
of promises;
I would have said yes
and meant it,
the roller coasters
I refused to ride
a poor imitation of the loop-d-loops
we face together.

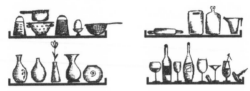

Chapter 11

Healthy, Wealthy, and Wise

This is what Alzheimer's does: Alzheimer's is a progressive brain disease in which abnormal protein deposits build up in the synapses causing cells to die which interrupts communication within the brain and creates problems with memory, thinking and behavior. As the disease develops, the more immediate memories—what day it is, what you had for breakfast, the name of the president of the United States—slip away, leaving only long-term memories intact. Eventually, patients lose the ability to recognize their loved ones; their appetite decreases; they forget basic skills; they become incontinent; they need assistance to eat, walk, dress, and more; they stop communicating; and they eventually become comatose.

According to the Center for Disease Control and Prevention, Alzheimer's is the sixth leading cause of death in the US.[18] It is thought, however, that many more deaths assigned to pneumonia, asphyxiation, general infection or even cardiac arrest, are actually complications from Alzheimer's.[19]

End stage Alzheimer's lasts one and a half to two years on average, according to the NIH.[20] I'm not sure that it's worth worrying about what actually kills you by the time you're at the end. The bigger issue is to make your loved one as comfortable as possible without needlessly extending their suffering.

It seems like a contradiction to say that in general Mom is healthy. But she is. That doesn't mean that her health won't slip or that we shouldn't monitor it. Mom has been subjected to doctor's visits, blood tests, urine tests, ultra sounds, even a mammogram. We have nursed her through her share of colds, fevers, and the dreaded UTI (urinary tract infection).

Each time we go back to the clinic, I weigh the significance of the test or procedure to be done not only in terms of its importance to mapping Mom's health but also to my ability to cajole, persuade, wheedle, charm or even bully Mom into doing something she is disinclined and/or incapable of doing.

The last time Mom had a mammogram was in 2014. She'd had a mammography test before, but she didn't remember what the procedure was or why she had to have one.

---

[18] Center for Disease Control and Prevention, "Leading Causes of Death," United States Health, 2016 (data from 2015).

[19] Blaszczak-Boxe, Agata, "Alzheimer's May Contribute to More Deaths than Thought," *Live Science,* March 5, 2014.

[20] National Institute on Aging, US Department of Health & Human Services, "End-of-Life Care for People with Dementia," May 17, 2017.

For those not in the know, a woman's breasts are X-rayed while she is in a standing position. The machine squeezes—the technical term is "compresses"—the breasts, one at a time, between two plates to create a flattened, round image of the breast tissue. And let me tell you, that compression hurts.

Mom was embarrassed about getting undressed. I persuaded her to take off her shirt and her bra and give me her long gold necklace to hold. The technician allowed me to stay inside with her for each of the four X-rays that were taken, slipping behind the barrier when the X-ray was in progress.

"I thought torture ended in the dark ages," Mom joked angrily when we were waiting for the disc containing her X-rays. "What was the point of that? I'm sorry you had to waste your time being here with me. I'm never doing that again."

"Ve have vays of making you talk," I whispered in my best German accent, getting at least a snort out of her.

I agreed. No more mammograms. Too painful.

In the winter of 2016, Mom contracted a UTI. We didn't know what was wrong. All we knew was that Mom had started complaining of tiredness and pains. Her abilities seemed to be in free fall. She was much more confused, dizzy and agitated. The standard symptoms of pain during urination were absent. Instead, it was as if her Alzheimer's symptoms were magnified.

Alzheimer's patients are prone to UTIs because they forget how to clean themselves well after going to the bathroom. Women are more susceptible to UTIs than men because women have shorter urethras and germs travel easily into the bladder and kidneys. Two for two.

Mom couldn't recognize what was happening to her body, let alone request help. She lay awake in bed one night shivering and shaking, and it was only by chance that Daddy woke up to find her. She was suddenly uttering nonsensical statements, searching for things that didn't exist, walking at a snail's pace and sleeping practically the whole day.

As a follow-up to her doctor's visit, the doctor sent us for a chest X-ray, urine and blood tests. I told Daddy I would take care of the X-ray and blood tests, but he'd have to manage to get the urine sample as I wouldn't arrive early enough in the morning to catch her first morning elimination. I also couldn't fathom how he'd get her to pee in a cup.

It was extremely difficult to convince Mom to cooperate. I could only imagine what it was like from her perspective. We pushed her to do uncomfortable things. To complete the X-ray, Mom had to undress and expose herself to the technician then take off her necklaces that she always wears and hand them to me. The technician showed her how she had to hug the machine in an embrace so that her body was flush against it, but the screen was cold. Closer, he admonished, closer. I can't count the number of times the work "f-ck" spewed from Mom's mouth, her face clenched in anger. Then she had to breathe in deeply and hold that breath without moving while the technician pressed a button. Shivering from cold and humiliation, Mom allowed me to assist her in redressing.

And blood tests: I thought they'd be easier. They seemed more manageable. They were an easy way to check the functioning of her internal organs. All she had to do was present her veins to the nurse. Granted, the nurse would probe her veins then tighten a tourniquet on her arm. But I would be there as she gazed with shock at the needle in the nurse's hands. I could make silly faces at her so that she wouldn't focus on that red liquid filling the test tubes. I could sing with her while she swore at everyone who passed and said I'd lied about it not being painful.

That's not even close to what happened.

We got to the clinic, took a number, and sang a few songs while we waited for our turn with the nurse. I joked with Mom that we were visiting vampires who required a taste of blood. Finally, our number was called. As Mom sat down at the nurse's station, I whispered to the nurse that Mom had Alzheimer's and suggested she reach out to Mom.

The nurse was patient and friendly. But Mom refused to show the nurse her arms. It wasn't like Mom was talking so coherently, but there were absolute moments of clarity when she knew what she was saying.

"I'm a real person," she announced. "I'm a proper person. And I don't like people talking about me."

Strike one.

"I don't share my blood with anyone," she declared a few minutes later.

Strike two.

We had been in this exact situation before, but previously Mom had been compliant. In fact, once, when I took her for an ultrasound, she lay on the table singing, "I've got you under my skin," which was so funny that we both laughed, and the nurse had to ask her to lie still.

This was different. I don't think Mom understood what was being asked of her, but she knew enough to refuse to cooperate with us. She may have even misunderstood what blood was.

Many words have lost their meaning. When she got dressed in the mornings, she couldn't distinguish between skirt, shirt, bra. When she was in the shower, she didn't know what soap was. She alternated between anger at being told the obvious ("Of course I've washed my face.

What do you take me for, an imbecile?"), and absolute incomprehension at the task before her.

"I am not interested in what you have to say. Today is not my time to give blood."

Strike three.

I looked at the nurse. How important were the blood tests? Could we wait and get them another day? I realized that there was nothing we could do or say—apart from physically forcing her—that would make Mom change her mind.

"Okay, that's it," I said. "We're leaving now."

Even in the midst of her obstinate mood, Mom accepted with alacrity the nurse's farewell wishes.

We went back to the waiting room and had a cool drink of water. Several minutes passed and I again told Mom that we had to get some blood tests done. Nope. It didn't make any dent in her intransigence.

I made the right decision by not forcing the issue. I just wonder if I could have done or said something differently that would have persuaded Mom to cooperate. Given my failure to produce blood samples, Daddy took Mom back to the clinic the next day and without a fuss she held out her arms to the nurse. I hold out hope that next time I can be more persuasive.

After the non-tests, we walked a few blocks to the nearby mall for a cup of coffee, but the short walk tired her out. Mom complained of feeling ill. She couldn't tell me more than that. No nausea. No dizziness. "Where does it hurt?" I asked.

She just didn't feel well, she didn't feel herself, and as she insistently told me, she was sorry I had to put up with her like that. We drank our coffee, then called Daddy to pick us up because the walk home was much too far for her. This was a walk we'd done hundreds of times. I was not sure when we would walk it again, if ever.

I tucked Mom into bed for her afternoon nap. She needed to sleep, she told me. Then, "I'm so glad I have you. We're so lucky to have each other, really."

Yes, I whispered. *I'm so glad you had me, too, because there is no place I'd rather be than by your side.*

By the time the UTI was diagnosed, Mom was on her second of three courses of anti-biotics. As the pills became difficult to swallow, we started dissolving them in cranberry juice.

Still, it would not go away. Mom was angry, bitter, depressed, and in pain. There were episodes where she described a burning sensation all over her body and yelled such hate-filled expletives. These were sometimes directed at us but most often toward herself.

My brother Simon came to visit during this illness. We took turns with Mom so that we shared the burden of her care. I was on call in the mornings to assist with showering and dressing, while Simon helped in the evenings.

Nighttime was especially difficult. What if Mom needed to get up and use the toilet while we were all sleeping? Could she find her way there? Could she find her way back to bed? We left the lights on where possible. Unfortunately, we hadn't thought to tape the sliding bolt on the door so that Mom wouldn't inadvertently lock herself in. Sure enough I awoke to hear her knocking and banging inside the bathroom hysterically trying to get out. We were just about to take the hinge off the door when somehow she managed to slide the bolt back. What relief we all felt when she opened the door.

As her health improved, I was grateful to realize Mom was returning to her previous level of cognitive ability. That meant, though, that she would once again block us from helping her when she went to the bathroom. She was still aware enough to demand privacy, and conversely, incapable of understanding our warnings about healthy bathroom habits.

We decided to take some precautions to reduce the risks of future UTIs. We would continue to give her a daily drink of cranberry juice and water, cranberry in pill form, and vitamin C. We made sure she emptied her bladder at two-to-three hour intervals (though this wasn't hard as Mom used the toiled frequently, often when she was bored). And we tried to persuade her to wash herself all over when she took her daily showers. Daddy also removed the bathroom lock so that Mom couldn't inadvertently lock herself in. Instead, he hung a sign on the bathroom door that could be flipped to read, "Occupied."

Dealing with Mom's illness felt as if we were barreling down a path strewn with rocky challenges. I much preferred the alternative—plodding along a rutted road going nowhere. Mom's recovery made me grateful that she could function at all. I blessed and cursed the future in equal measures knowing how hard it would be to deal with Mom as she slid cognitively. What would I do when I could no longer feed my craving for the genuine laughter and joy that she was still capable of sharing with us?

ၜၜ

It was the advertisement for the red toilet seat that caught my attention. What's with that, I wondered, and why is it appearing on an Alzheimer's website alongside red plates, red utensils, red handrails, red...well, you name it.

Our eyes are apparently expert at seeing red. Of the six to seven million cones in the retina—tiny cells that respond to light—about sixty-four percent respond most strongly to red light, while about a third are set off the most by green light, and another two percent respond to blue light.[21]

While Alzheimer's patients' eyes might register in an eye exam as being just fine, their capacity to "see" is often affected in practice. Not only does the ability to discern depth disappear, but so does color perception. As our eyes age, many of us lose some aptitude in judging between colors; people with Alzheimer's seem to experience a greater loss. Apparently, their greatest difficulty lies in differentiating colors in the blue-violet spectrum, while red is the easiest color for them to perceive.[22]

So imagine you open the white door to your white and beige bathroom, to be greeted by a white tiled floor, beige counters, beige towels on the rack, and a white toilet. The toilet effectively disappears.

What if this understanding of vision played a role in Alzheimer's patient's reluctance to eat? This phenomenon was tested by Boston University bio-psychologist Alice Cronin-Golomb and her research partners who published an article in 2004 subtitled, "If You Couldn't See Your Mashed Potatoes, You Probably Wouldn't Eat Them."[23]

According to Dr. Cronin-Golomb, staff in nursing homes complained that patients with Alzheimer's did not finish the food on their plates even when the staff encouraged them to eat. Weight loss in Alzheimer's patients—up to forty percent lose an unhealthy amount of weight—has been attributed to depression, the inability to concen-

[21] Pappas, Stephanie, "How We See Color," *Live Science,* April 29, 2010

[22] "The Alzheimer's Eye Sees Things Differently," The Eldercare Team, January 11, 2013

[23] Schwab, Jeremy, "Out of Sight, Out of Mind: If You Couldn't See Your Mashed Potatoes, You Probably Wouldn't Eat Them," *Arts & Sciences Magazine,* Boston University, Spring 2010.

trate on more than one food on their plate at a time, even on the inability to eat unassisted. But when Cronin-Golomb's team tested advanced Alzheimer's patients' level of food intake with not only standard white plates but also bright red ones, they discovered that patients eating from red plates consumed twenty-five percent more food than those eating from white plates.[24]

With research like the "red plate experiment," we can make things easier for Alzheimer's patients as their cognitive abilities decline. Mom, however, may not need to eat more than she already does, regardless of the plate's color, as she's actually gained a lot of weight recently.

With my thoughts focused on the color red, I began to notice red things all around me: the red playground near my house, a red gym bag, my red shopping wagon, red vegetables, red shoes, red stripes on my daughter's sheets. How will we know when Mom is ready for red plates and red toilet seats? Many aspects of this disease are so subtle—the downward slide occurring imperceptibly—that we may not know.

I'm open to buying some red plates. The toilet seat? I'm still working on accepting that idea.

ে৯৫৯

Color is an important factor in how appetizing food is. In the tomato, color is wedded to a wholesome source of antioxidants, lycopene and other nutrients. Some studies say that antioxidants can reduce the risk of Alzheimer's, while lycopene fights heart disease. Notwith-

---

[24] Ibid.

standing my love for the book, *Fried Green Tomatoes*,[25] here are three recipes that use red tomatoes as a main ingredient.

---

[25] Flag, Fannie, *Fried Green Tomatoes at the Whistle Stop Café,* Random House, USA, 1987

Roasted Tomatoes with Parsley and Garlic

A recipe for when tomatoes are plentiful. It's easy to make and will impress your guests with its elegance. Dare to make more than just the amount listed below, especially if you are a tomato lover.

5 tomatoes, halved
Olive oil
3-4 cloves garlic, finely chopped
½ cup fresh parsley, chopped
Sea salt and pepper to taste

Directions:
Halve tomatoes and place in a baking dish cut side up. Liberally brush each tomato with olive oil. Sprinkle with chopped garlic, large-grained salt, pepper and parsley. Roast at 350 degrees F / 180 degrees C for thirty to forty minutes. Serve warm.

Pesto Pizza

This is an alternative to pizza if you are lactose intolerant like my dad. Try it with red peppers and onions, olives, or a combination of vegetables. Hat tip to Susie Fishbein's Kosher by Design.[26]

Crust:
1½ cups flour
½ cup canola oil
5 Tbsp cold water
1 tsp salt

Pesto:
1 cup fresh basil leaves
3 cloves garlic
¼ cup pine nuts (or walnuts)
⅓ cup olive oil
1 Tbsp mayonnaise
Salt and pepper to taste

Toppings:
2 to 3 large tomatoes sliced
Salt and pepper

Directions:
Preheat oven to 350 degrees F / 180 degrees C. In a small bowl, mix crust. Pat dough into a nine-inch / twenty-three-cm pie pan, and up the sides. Bake pie crust for fifteen minutes. Remove and let cool. Meanwhile, combine pesto ingredients in a food processor. Spoon pesto into cooled pie pan, top with sliced tomatoes, sprinkle with salt and pepper and bake an additional fifteen minutes.

---

[26] Fishbein, Susie, *Kosher by Design Short on Time,* Artscroll/Shaar Press, New York, 2006

Shakshuka

This breakfast dish is apparently of Libyan origin and is served all day at most cafés in Israel. The basic ingredients are eggs and tomatoes. If I'm making shakshuka for the whole family, I'll prepare two pans at once, or one pan with five or six eggs, doubling the amount of crushed tomatoes and paste I use.

1 Tbsp olive oil
1-2 cloves crushed garlic
1 small onion chopped
1 red pepper chopped
1 cup crushed tomatoes
2 Tbsp tomato paste
2-3 eggs
½ tsp cumin
¼ cup parmesan cheese, grated
Salt and pepper to taste

Directions:
In a small frying pan, sauté garlic and onion in oil until onion becomes translucent. Add pepper and spices. Stir. Add tomatoes and tomato paste. Stir and simmer for about ten minutes. Make two (or three) small indentations in the sauce with a spoon and break eggs into these shallow holes, keeping the yolk whole. Simmer covered up to twenty minutes until eggs cook. Sprinkle with cheese and remove from flame.

Onions

It gives me pleasure to cut you,
to crumple your brown skin
and expose your white eternity,
circles within circles like the onions
entombed in Ramses' eye sockets.
My ancestors longed for you
when they left Egypt.

Other people cry over you, but not me.
I chop, pare, peel, slice, dice
my way through your sharp curves.

Once, for a school experiment,
we rested you in a cup of water
and watched you sprout pale green shoots.
I almost loved you then.

How sweet you are when I plunge you
into burning coals in the barbecue.
Pliny the Elder believed you healed
mouth sores, dog bites and tooth aches,
that your bitter taste induced sleep.

I keep you hidden under my sink,
take you out when I need you,
wipe your milky blood from my counters.
I give you voice
when you sizzle in my pan.

Chapter 12

Happy Holidays, Trying Times

Caring for someone with Alzheimer's is like working in the dark. It is hard to know how to respond to some of the situations that Mom presents. Often, I am left feeling guilty that I haven't done enough. Or there's the nagging sense that I'm not a talented enough caregiver in reducing the anger that flares so suddenly.

Mom sounded so *normal* on the phone when I invited her to celebrate Purim with us in 2017. This is the holiday when we read the story of Esther saving the Jews of Persia from execution.

"We'd love to come visit you!" she beamed.

Of course, the moment I opened the door to my house to invite them inside, Mom looked at me, puzzled, and declared, "I didn't know you lived here."

I laughed. I had been feeling anxious about their visit, about all I needed to do, all that could go wrong, the energy I'd need to entertain them. Here we were on the threshold, literally and figuratively, and I had a choice to make. I could continue to run scenarios in my head about how this visit would go or I could be in the moment. I made up my mind to sweep away the dread that had been gathering inside me and, as best I could, enter into her world.

That Purim visit actually went quite well. Mom agreed to wear a witch's hat as dress-up and proceeded to entertain us with her most scary witch's cackle. When we attended our synagogue's communal meal, I could see she was overwhelmed by the number of people around her, the noise, even the food choices. She didn't recognize anyone, not even my in-laws who were visiting from the States, but she hid it well and graciously talked to everyone who came by to say hello.

As usual, the fun started when Mom had to get ready for bed. At first, she was frantically looking for something, a specific paper or other imaginary object that she felt was missing. I finally gave her a small piece of paper and a pencil. She wrote a note to herself—with our assistance as she desperately searched for the words to an unknown yet urgent message—which seemed to greatly calm her:

MIRIA'M'S BE'R SHE
VER
Check with JACK
MARCH 12
END OF PURIM
LUV, NA

I guess this was a message to remind her that she was at my house, her precious husband was with her, and the holiday of Purim was over. As a final touch, as it was a note to herself, she added "Love, Na" (Na being short for Naomi).

Daddy persuaded her to undress for bed. Then she

insisted that she needed her shoes so that she could go home. I could hear their voices being raised as Daddy tried to rationally explain that they were staying over for the night. It had been a full, active day, and all I wanted was to go to sleep. I knocked on their door and suggested Mom come sit with me in the living room. My husband Jeff put on some slow melodious torch songs, and we sat and sang along for about ten minutes. This calmed both of us, and I was able to lead her happily back to her room. She climbed into bed and easily fell asleep.

When Passover rolled around just one month later, I again invited my parents to celebrate with us. Seder is a magical night for most Jewish families as it celebrates the exodus from Egypt that is written about extensively in the Torah.

This time, on the eve of their arrival, I wrote myself a list of things I could do to reduce the stress.

* *Make signs that list what's in the kitchen cabinets.* Maybe this will help Mom remember where we've put things for Passover as we switch many of our dishes and food items from their regular cabinets.

* *Tape the lock in the bathroom so it can't be used.* Mom had locked herself in the bathroom on several occasions in my home and in her own home, and her panic was palpable. The last time it happened, I really thought we'd have to break down the door to get her out. Shockingly, she somehow managed to open it by herself. I don't want to go through that again.

* *Cook as much as I can before my parents arrive.* I'd rather dedicate my attention to Mom than to tasks in the kitchen, if I can help it.

* Devise simple tasks for Mom to assist with. Meaning, if I don't accomplish the previous items well enough, I have to figure out how to keep Mom occupied while I finish up my cooking.

* Give my kids a pep talk. My kids used to have the most interactive grandmother around, one who would get down on the floor and play with them, read to them, and sing to them. She can't do that anymore. And she often isn't the sweet-natured woman she once was. I want to help them connect to her on her current level. I have been planning on bringing out some of the books they used to love as kids in the hope that they would now read them to her.

* Note to self: Relax. Remember to sing. Prepare for the unpredictable. Don't try to always be in control. Delegate. Enjoy. Love. Breathe.

My feeling is that there is no magic in finding a path through the maze that is Alzheimer's. There is only trial and error, tuning into the person you are caring for and finding the best and most positive solution possible at any given moment.

I'm not sure how I find the creativity and patience to be with Mom, but I am content that I am able to contribute in some small way to her happiness.

When she was with us on these extended family get-togethers, I knew that I was not alone in caring for Mom. She was with people who truly loved her. What could go wrong?

Those famous last words.

ฆฆฆ

This past winter, as I was taking Mom home from a Chanukah sing-a-long, I lost my temper. Mom had taken my coat and wouldn't give it back. The moment I yelled at her, though, I regretted it terribly.

Here's what transpired: We had attended a sing-a-long of Chanukah songs. About an hour into enjoying the music and humming along to most of the songs, Mom asked me to find her coat so that she could put it on. Then she saw another coat on the back of a chair near her and wanted to put that one on, too.

"That's not your coat," I tried to explain. "You have your coat on. That coat belongs to someone else."

"Give me my coat," she thundered. "That's mine. Why won't you let me take my suitcase?"

Suitcase? Mom had been talking sweetly all evening in a free-flowing way, mostly making no sense, but she'd been in a good mood. Now we were at the precipice of a melt down and we needed to move on.

In order to prevent her from taking that other coat, I handed her mine. It's only a five minute walk back to her house, I reasoned. How cold could it be?

I don't know if I can sufficiently convey the absurd nature of our interaction. Mom begrudgingly took my proffered coat, zippered it up over her other three layers, then walked with me toward her home, grumbling all the way. It was as if she didn't trust me to take her the right way and she questioned every step we took.

It *was* chilly outside.

"Don't be absurd," she barked when I asked for my coat back. "You should have thought of that before, you silly girl."

Okay, I thought, *I'll just wait until I get her home.* She'll have to take it off then. I sang one of the songs from the sing-a-long over and over to keep us moving forward.

Finally we reached her door.

The moment she stepped inside her house, I asked her for my coat.

"This is mine!" she shouted. "I won't give this to you!"

"Give me back my coat," I shouted back, my frustration blazing without warning.

"Naomi," my dad responded, "this is not your coat." Daddy had not come with us.

"What do you mean it's not my coat? How dare you talk to me like that? Apologize to me this instance!" Mom exploded. "Apologize!"

Mom was inches from his face, her anger palpable, her skin turning bright red.

Oh, no, I thought, *what have I done?*

By this time, Daddy had maneuvered Mom out of not only my coat but her own coat and was leading her to their bedroom to undress for the night. Holding the coat behind my back, I sincerely apologized to Mom for making her so upset.

"I should hope so," she countered as she moved away, railing all the while against Daddy's ministrations.

When they entered their room and shut the door, I slipped out and started for home. I felt like I was abandoning my post, but I also realized that my presence was not needed.

As emotional as I felt, I started to analyze the situation. Here are three observations I made during this incident.

1. Mom's transition from calm sweetness to an irrational ogre happened abruptly. This may be part of the larger pattern that has been developing these last few weeks. Our caretaker Sahlee has noticed that when Mom

wears her Exelon[27] patch—a medicine the doctor has suggested we stop giving her—she is more even-keeled. But this, too, has a limited effectiveness; we must be prepared for more sudden uncontrolled outbursts.

2 I have to do a better job of controlling my own emotions. I might not like Mom's anger, but I'm in a position to control my moods, while she's not.

3. My dad is possibly more adept than I am at working through Mom's mood swings. His use of logic is lost on Mom, but she listens to him. I must bow to his greater influence.

I got my coat back, but I felt sheepish. My noble plan to give my dad an extra break by taking Mom to the sing-a-long almost backfired. Thankfully his sensibilities prevailed in dealing with Mom's intransigence.

And days later I was still troubled by my behavior. How could I have let myself get so emotional over a *damned coat*? Perhaps I should have asked to borrow the coat that had been hanging on the back of the chair. I could have let Mom wear it home then brought it back to its owner.

Or I could have insisted that she listen to me.

Actually, I know I couldn't do that. It would have meant forcing her to accept my reality. And if there's anything I've learned, it's that with Alzheimer's patients, reality is subjective. Mom's perception of the world is usually sweetly colored, but sometimes the world is an unpredictably black place.

---

[27] Exelon (Rivastigmine, Aricept) is used to treat mild to moderate dementia caused by Alzheimer's or Parkinson's disease. It prevents the breakdown of a chemical in the memory, thinking and reasoning processes.

Mom doesn't remember anything of this incident. It's time for me to move on, too.

‿౿‿

The fact that I am sometimes unable to keep Mom calm depresses me. What can I do differently? The Alzheimer's-focused websites give suggestions as to how to avoid confrontation, for example, when Mom stands in her own living room and says she must go home. Comfort her, is one suggestion. But I am left with many questions. What is she really asking? Where does her anxiety to go "home" stem from? Is there a way to distract her from her single-minded pursuit?

My fear is that these are all one-time solutions to issues that recur with greater frequency the longer Mom suffers from this disease. When we go out for coffee, Mom suddenly decides it is time to leave and bolts from the table. How can I stop her? Must I physically stand in her way? How do I communicate with her if she's in such a blustery, angry state? Is there another way?

I have recently finished reading a book called *Contented Dementia: 24-Hour Wraparound Care for Lifelong Well-being*[28] that was suggested by a friend. This book speaks my language. It puts into a framework of caring for dementia patients many of the ways I've tried to interact with Mom. It does it in a concrete way that gives expression to and formalizes the way we interact. I don't believe it can solve all our problems, but I'm willing to give it a try.

The author writes about his mother-in-law, Penny Garner, and her many years of volunteering with Alz-

---

[28] James, Oliver, *Contented Dementia: 24-Hour Wraparound Care for Lifelong Well-being*, Vermillion, London, 2008

heimer's patients, first with her mother and then in the British health care system, to create a program called SPECAL, Specialized Early Care for Alzheimer's (pronounced like "special").

Garner uses the analogy of a photograph album to explain how normal memory works, what happens as we age, and the single dramatic change which occurs with the onset of dementia. The photo album represents our memory system, with individual memories symbolized by individual photographs. With normal memory everything that has just happened in our life is stored, unconsciously, moment by moment, as photographs in our album that record facts and associated feelings of an event. We use our album as a crucial reference point to provide context in our life. As we age, we continue to store photographs in the normal way but we become slower at accessing the information that we need. It is there, but sometimes it takes us so long to find that it is no longer useful to us, for example, we want to reference a person's name but the photograph of that individual becomes inaccessible.

With the onset of dementia there is a crucial process change: a new type of photograph containing feelings but no facts enters the album. The book calls this new type of photograph a "blank." For Mom, it's as if the conversation I had with her half an hour ago never happened or the songs we sang while sitting on the couch were never sung. I might have a snapshot of them in my own album, but in Mom's album the photographs are increasingly lacking in facts, with just the feelings present. If challenged on a specific memory (like telling Mom she can't eat lunch because she's already had lunch), Mom would not be able to find photographs reflecting this; she would therefore not reconcile a dirty plate sitting in the sink as evidence that she had had lunch—and my disagreement with her own record of recent events would lead to panic and self-doubt at not being able to remember the simplest of events—at having a black, gaping hole where her memory should be—namely having eaten lunch.

The photographs of our disagreement over whether she had eaten lunch might be blank in terms of facts, but the feelings will be stored, providing her with unexplained distress, anxiety, anger, or fear, which can destroy the daily well-being of the individual. I know for a fact that Mom is aware of her memory loss. She has told me so on numerous occasions and it distresses her to realize she can no longer recall things. This would be enough to send me into a panic, as it does her.

Drama and trauma do resonate much more strongly with Alzheimer's patients, precisely because the album is becoming less cluttered with facts. I remember, once, spilling my coffee when Mom and I were out together. Whatever else happened that day is gone, but the immediate concern that Mom conjured up—the worry, the fuss, the disquiet—that I might be hurt or burnt affected her in ways that other more placid events did not.

And of our time together that day, her reaction stays with me.

There is much to be praised in this SPECAL care method. I particularly like the three cardinal rules:

* Rule no. 1: Don't ask direct questions.

There are too many variables in answering a question if your album pages are filling up with blanks. For example, if I am asked, "Do you want a cup of coffee?" I have to reference in my album whether I've had one, or if there's milk, or time, or some without caffeine. Better to say to Mom, "I think it's a good time to have a cup of coffee," leaving her the option of joining in or not, without putting her on the spot with a direct question.

* Rule No. 2: Learn from the experts.

If we are keyed in to Mom's verbal and body language, she can teach us words and phrases, gestures and movements that make sense to her, drawn largely from the pre-dementia pages in her album. We need to listen and learn from her and use her language ourselves as it will make far more sense to her.

* Rule no. 3: Never contradict.

To alleviate negative clashes, Garner suggests avoiding direct contradiction, knowing that the person is using their own album in the way that works best for them, often using facts from pages way back in the album rather than the more recent "blank" photos. As a caregiver who is in control of her facilities, responding in a non-confrontational manner to convey the sense that the dementia patient was right ("You're right, I was mistaken."), ensures that the conflict never escalates into those strong emotions, and the individual maintains her sense of coherence and well-being.

To be in a state of constantly questioning our sense of reality—to have blank pages in our album—can lessen our sense of self-worth and our equilibrium. Our goal as caregivers, according to SPECAL, is to return that sense of self to our loved ones.

When my husband Jeff and I started arguing about whether he had or had not told me about the lecture he was planning to attend, I realized that I was experiencing on a small scale what Mom experienced every day. I could not remember having been told. The information was utterly gone, and I refused to believe that Jeff had conveyed the information. We would have been in much better shape if one of us had had the alacrity to state, "silly me, you're right, you did tell me," or, "you're right, I forgot to tell you." All argument would have ceased, and regardless of the correct version of events, our competing egos would have been soothed.

When we are missing the facts of recent events, we go in search of past photographs to provide context. We flip through our album to find memories that seem to match what we see or feel today. The *Contented Dementia* book describes one woman with dementia who had always been an avid traveler as referencing her many early memories of traveling whenever she was in a situation with people around her, such as a doctor's office. When she asked her companion if their bags had been checked, an answer that alludes to an airport situation would calm her. What appears from the outside to be strange, possibly hallucinatory language, is actually somewhat logical. But if the travel scenario is broken, the woman can lose her sense of coherence and become hostile or anxious out of fear of not understanding where she is.

The book has exercises to follow—homework, if you will—to help us understand the person we are caring for. We must listen to Mom and see what she can tell us about herself. With a little sleuthing—considering her thought process and language is often quite bizarre—we might be able to connect a past experience from her photo album which she is using to make sense of what she is doing now in the present.

芝芝芝

If I examine past interactions with Mom within the lens of the SPECAL method, I realize I've been on the right track all along. I just haven't had the framework or language to develop my care of Mom further.

I knew we were at a crossroads when we had to decide whether or not to give Mom anti-psychotic medication to combat her hostility and irrational behavior (i.e., hallucinations, delusions, aggression, agitation, and un-cooperativeness,), thereby knowingly embracing possible side-effects of these drugs. The alternative, or so it seemed, was to continue to shepherd Mom through her heart breaking performances and embrace her anger.

The use of anti-psychotic drugs must be considered with extreme caution. No drugs are specifically approved by the US Food and Drug Administration to treat behavioral and psychiatric dementia symptoms in Alzheimer's patients, though "off label" use, where a doctor prescribes a drug for a different purpose than the one for which it is approved, is an accepted practice. How much is too much agitation? What defines a hallucination? Are there other alternatives? What are the risks involved? Is Mom a danger to herself? Who are the drugs really for—her or us?

We knew from past experience that even on a very low dose of one of the recommended drugs, Mom's gait slowed significantly, she slept more, and her speech became more incoherent. But she also seemed more compliant and generally happy.

My dad is the one who spends all day every day with Mom. He has little time for himself, and he is often in conflict with Mom over her behavior. I had a renewed sense of his experience when he was out of the house for the whole day, and I was the key caregiver.

Several times during the day, Mom told me she had to leave. She walked to the back of the house and went from one room to the other in a desperate search for a way to the non-existent upstairs floors. In one room, she went into the corner and dramatically pressed along the wall as if looking for a secret passageway. Back in the hall, she fumbled with the door, trying to figure out how to open it. Then she went into the study, stood by the desk examining what was on it, opened the file drawer, and rummaged through it. I walked with her on several of her circuits, surprised at one point to find a folded manila folder under her skirt.

It was only eight a.m. the first time she walked this circuit, too early to head to the local mall. I took the advice of our caregiver Sahlee and let Mom struggle on her own. If we didn't talk to her, she seemed less angry. But I was heartbroken to watch her actions, knowing I could not help her or calm her in any way. When it was late enough to walk out, Mom hesitated. She told me she needed to stay where she was to find the way home. When I showed her the door at the other end of the apartment, she reluctantly followed me out.

In that instance, Mom's mood switched. We had a great time walking and talking, drinking coffee, window shopping, visiting rabbits in the pet shop, and commenting on the people around us. On our walk home, Mom continued to radiate happiness. When we arrived, we made doughnuts for Chanukah. We listened to Benny Goodman, sat in the sunshine, swung our legs on the bed, and laughed about everything.

"This isn't my house," Mom said suddenly.

And so began Mom's second round of "going home." She refused to eat lunch. She refused to take her nap. We checked up on her occasionally, but our idea was that she'd eventually tire and want to sleep.

I asked Mom if she'd like to help me bake the doughnuts. No. Mom expressed an urgency to stay where she was.

I took Mom into her bedroom, thinking I could convince her to nap by lying down with her. Ha, ha. Mom examined everything in the room. She sat at the edge of the bed and made her skirt into a kind of pocket so that she could put things she'd gathered in it. Of course, the minute she stood up they all fell out. So she took off her skirt. She found a sweater and put it on over her other two layers. She took it off, put her skirt back on, then put on one of Daddy's sweaters.

She placed things under her pillow, including her purse, some tissues, a file from the computer room, and Daddy's sweat pants. All the while she kept up a running commentary on everything that she was doing. Most of it involved saying goodbye to me and kissing the top of my head because she was apparently heading off into the wild unknown.

Two hours later, we left her room. Sahlee got her to finally sit down, and then miraculously, her mood changed again. She ate lunch, had a cup of tea, talked and giggled, and somehow seemed to gain a modicum of normality. By then, thankfully, it was time to pick Daddy up at the train station.

What a greeting Daddy received. Here was Mom's sun returned to her.

"I bet you're glad I'm home," he quipped.

And I was.

As to the drugs, it was not my decision to make. But I guess you know how I felt. I didn't want to lose any part of Mom that could interact with us with joy and laughter.

The one incident that stands out in my mind as an all-time horrible experience occurred only a few weeks later. It was the straw that made me want to find a better way.

Mom attacked me. I am still trying to process our physical scuffle.

I thought we were being cruel by administering her anti-psychotic meds. It made her drowsy and slow, reduced her gait to a shuffle, and seemed to fuel her delusional ramblings. I had convinced Daddy to reduce the dose, but now I could see that it did have an effect on her. Yes, without it she had more stamina to walk, but her desire to "go home" returned with a vengeance. This is what caused her to physically fight me.

It started after a trip to the grocery store and a fruitless visit to the hairdresser. Mom was happy to greet the hairdresser, shake his hand, try his comfortable chair, but she was adamant that she could not stay. She told us she had places to be, and that she'd return to have her hair cut some other time. We walked around the block and back but it made no difference. So we headed for home.

Once we were home, Mom said right away she needed to leave. There were people waiting for her, she explained, and she was leaving whether I was ready or not. Sahlee, our caregiver, suggested we lock the door, but I, in my greater wisdom, thought that was cruel, too.

I told Sahlee I would take her for a walk. I figured we could sit on a bench in the sun as we'd done so many times before. I assumed it would be easy to steer her through the paths outside the house and bring her safely home.

The minute Mom got out the door, she turned left and headed straight down one particular path. She would not sit on the bench with me, even when I feigned dizziness. She would not stop to say hello to the kids in the local kindergarten. No, she was determined to walk that straight path to its end. I realized that I could not let her do that, because where the path ended, there was a muddy drop that she could not have navigated.

I stood in front of her and told her we had to turn around. I gave her choices, I raised my voice, I tried to physically turn her. She lashed out at me. She grabbed my arm and dug her fingernails into my skin. I wrapped my arms around her and hugged her as tightly as I could. She screamed for help, for the police, for God to take this evil woman away from her. She punched my chin. Somehow, when I let go, she stormed away from me in the right direction.

When we got back to her house, she almost escaped by unlocking the door when I wasn't looking. With Sahlee's help, we got her inside and locked the top lock on front door, which she rattled with great intensity but could not open.

Sahlee told her that only my dad had the key. To bide our time, I put on a movie and tried to entice her to sing with me. Thankfully, and to our great relief, Daddy came home around then. I noticed, though, that she was just as antsy with him as she had been with me. She again told us she had to leave, but he was able to defuse her mood.

By the time I left, Mom was happily singing with me and even gave me a kiss goodbye. Thank God she has no memory of her actions—or mine. It's bad enough that I have to relive how I treated her in those moments. I'm worried, though, that the strong emotions will linger on.

Taking the SPECAL method a step further can potentially allow Daddy and me to tailor a whole life style plan that includes ways to help gain Mom's trust, to wash her hair, go to the bathroom, visit a doctor's office, stay calm in the face of Daddy's absence, and even back down from extreme situations.

It revolves around careful observation to discover which of her old photographs are useful to Mom. It means listening to Mom talk, playing a verbal ping-pong with her, testing themes and gestures to see which ones are most useful to her. If we can identify the themes which resonate, we can link these to all the routine activities of daily life and make her days a series of benign repeating loops to create a fluid, calm environment.

I know that adding elements from the SPECAL method will improve not only Mom's emotional state but our own. It is an ongoing proposition to care for Mom as serenely as possible, one that fluctuates as the blanks gradually increase in her album. We will not see change overnight. Last month, on a particularly hot day, I was proud of myself for bringing Mom home from the mall with absolutely no display of anger. It was an intense effort to be with her and talk to her in a deferential, unquestioning manner. When she adamantly told me that the door in front of us was the door to her apartment, I did not stop her from knocking. Fortunately, she found it locked and allowed me to lead her to her own door. And if someone had answered, I would have improvised in as positive a manner as I could. I want to relinquish the guilt I feel when I am incapable of helping Mom out of her worrisome emotions and wrong turns. The SPECAL method helps me to do this.

೧೦೪೨

Being together as a three- and four-generational family is always special on the Jewish holidays. We eat well whether it is Rosh Hashanah, Chanukah, Purim, or Passover. Sweet and sour meatballs, roast chicken, potato kugel, carrot kugel, and many salads. Though visiting us in Beer Sheva is becoming increasingly difficult, as moving Mom from her home environment for even a few days creates all sorts of stress, Mom and Daddy still come stay with us most years on the three pilgrimage festivals: Sukkot, Passover and Shavuot. When my grandmother Millie was able to travel, she would join us, too. On more than one occasion, we conducted a four-generational Seder. One memorable Passover, with Simon and his wife Sharon visiting from California, the house bursting with relatives, Booba decided to take over the kitchen and make "bubalehs," a delightful almond and egg pancake. As a child, I always thought they were called bubalehs because Booba was the only one who could make them. I had tried numerous times without success. Simon managed to film her frying them, her batter-smeared fingers touching almost everything in my kitchen, creating havoc only she knew how to make. Here are several recipes, including the bubalehs and the doughnuts mentioned earlier that Mom helped me make, that grace our table on these wonderful family gatherings.

Bubalehs

The problem with this recipe is that my grandmother never used exact measurements. She just tossed ingredients into her bowl until it looked and felt right. I have been able to refine the amounts but there's still a give-and-take to this recipe that reminds me of her standing in my kitchen and making me peer into the bowl to see the batter's consistency. As soon as she'd finish frying a batch, we'd pester her to make more. Start with two eggs. This will make eight to ten small pancakes.

2 eggs
¾ cup ground almonds (approximate)
1 Tbsp sugar
1 Tbsp canola oil for frying (more if needed)
½ tsp vanilla (optional)
Sugar for dredging

Directions:
Whisk eggs until light and fluffy. Add incrementally sugar and almonds and continue whisking. Batter should be light yellow and not too thick. Heat oil in a non-stick frying pan. Using a table spoon, spoon batter into pan and fry on medium heat until edges begin to brown. Flip and continue frying. Remove from pan when browned on both sides and, still hot, dredge on a plate of granulated sugar. Eat immediately.

Maple Chicken with Carrots and Onions

When making this dish for Passover, it helps to have a daughter who has just returned from Montreal with a can of pure maple syrup in her suitcase, but I've also substituted imitation maple syrup and it works just fine.

14 chicken pieces with skin
8-10 carrots, cut into think sticks
1 onion, sliced

Sauce:
3 Tbsp olive oil
⅓ cup maple syrup
¾ cup brown sugar
1 Tbsp dried oregano
Salt and pepper to taste

Directions:
In a large pan, place chicken pieces in single layer in one part and the carrots and onions in another part. Rub sauce onto chicken pieces and sprinkle remaining sauce over vegetables. Cook for 45 minutes to an hour at 375 degrees F / 190 degrees C or until both chicken and carrots brown on top.

Passover Quiche

I enjoy eating dairy meals on Passover. It is a break from the traditional meat meals we eat on the first and last nights of the holiday. It also means I get to use the pretty once-a-year glass dishes my mother-in-law bought us when we were married. This is an adaptation of the quiche recipe I learned to bake when I was in college.

Crust:
4 whole matzot (plural of matza)
Filling:
1 onion sliced into rings
1 Tbsp oil
1½ cups grated cheese (try yellow cheese, or add some cheddar)

Custard:
4 eggs
1½ cups milk
1 Tbsp matza meal
¼ tsp salt
Paprika

Directions:
To make the matzas soft and bendable, take four whole matzas and wet them under water in the kitchen sink. Place them one by one on a large plate separated by soaking wet paper towels. Let sit for approximately twenty minutes. While you are waiting for the matzas to soften, fry onion rings in oil until they begin to brown. In a separate bowl, mix custard ingredients. Set aside. When matzas are soft, drape them in the nine-inch / twenty-three-cm quiche pan with four corners overlapping in the center (i.e., each matza is on a diagonal with one corner in the

middle of the pan), making sure to pat the matzas with your hands into the shape of the pan. You may cut the excess matza with a knife or scissors around the edge of the pan. Lay the cheese on top of the matza crust. Spread out the onions. Pour custard on top. Top with a sprinkling of paprika. Bake at 350 degrees F / 180 degrees C for forty-five minutes.

Saba No-Fry Doughnuts

I made these doughnuts specifically for my dad—no milk, no fried dough. They came out well; they give the illusion of eating a doughnut. The less you knead the dough, the spongier the doughnuts.

2 tsp yeast
½ cup sugar
¾ cup warm soy milk
4 eggs
½ cup oil
3¾ cups flour
1 tsp salt
1 tsp vanilla

Icing: (for chocolate icing add 2½ Tbsp baking cocoa)
1½ cups powdered sugar
2-3 Tbsp soy milk
1½ tsp vanilla

Directions:
Proof yeast in a bowl by adding, sugar and warm soy milk. Let react for fifteen minutes. Add eggs and vanilla, flour and salt. Knead till dough forms. Let rise for two hours. Refrigerate dough for at least an hour (can be up to two days). Remove from fridge and without kneading, grab a fist-sized chunk of dough and wrap around a small, round cookie cutter or other item to make a doughnut hole. Place on baking tray. When all doughnuts are made, cover and let rise for up to an hour in a warm area. Brush tops with egg and bake at 375 degrees F / 190 degrees C for fifteen minutes. In a separate bowl, mix icing ingredients. Dip warm doughnuts in icing then let cool. Microwave for fifteen seconds just before eating.

Frog in My Throat

I tell her there's a frog in my throat.
She believes me.
I wanted to humor her,
but she's asking how it got there
and do I need her help to get it out.

We sing the song she taught me,
frogs jumping on Pharaoh's bed and head,
on his toes and nose.
We laugh together.
Then she tells me, "I found my nose.
I have noses.
I have husbands with noses."

I'm writing a new song
for the two of us.
It's filled with sparkling laughter
and an uncommon love
for the mother as child,
for the daughter she no longer recognizes.

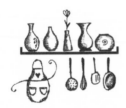
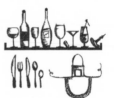

Chapter 13

Honor Thy Mother

*D*on't worry, it'll get easier. That's the advice several well-meaning friends gave me. I wanted to ask: *How? Will it get easier when she needs help every time she goes to the bathroom or when she can't dress herself? Will it get easier when her last hold on reality slips away and she doesn't know me at all?* Some advice. I didn't know how to react.

Then I spoke to Drora.

Every week I watched as Drora and her mom, Aliza, entered our synagogue. I'd seen Aliza progress from a well-dressed, inquisitive woman to a wheelchair-bound thin-faced invalid. How could that be *easier*? Drora's mom could no longer stand. She barely recognized her own granddaughters. She mostly stared straight ahead into emptiness. Drora fussed over her mother with care. When Aliza's body slowly bent forward, Drora would matter-of-factly push her back into a sitting position. She'd smooth her mom's hair, listen to her whispered ramblings, and hold her hand. This was courageous love, a true honoring of one's parent.

"How can it possibly get easier?" I asked Drora one Saturday afternoon. "I'm expecting only the worst."

"It *does*," Drora told me earnestly. "It gets easier when they become more pliant and stop fighting you."

Immediately, I thought of Mom's temper flares, the way she fought us when we suggested she wear something more appropriate, the agitation she felt at not understanding conversations or feeling left out. I thought of the argument she and Daddy had when he mentioned a film they'd watched, and she adamantly denied ever having watched it, screaming at him for lying. I thought of all the times she denigrated herself with horrible swear words over misplaced items or misunderstood instructions. And I knew Drora was right. In a perverse way, it would get better as it got worse.

When Drora's mom, Aliza, passed away at the age of eighty-seven after a seven-year battle with Alzheimer's, I cried for Drora. Aliza spent her last week in the hospital comatose, unable to eat or drink or understand anything that was happening around her. She had become a hollow shell of the person she once was, and it was our job to help Drora remember her as she used to be.

When I thought of my own mother battling the same killer, when I watched her strange behavior—putting on three skirts when she got dressed, pouring bleach in the washer instead of detergent, thinking I'm her sister—I ached for what Drora was going through. My goal was to spend as much time with Mom as I could, and, when she forgot who I was, to hope that Mom's emotional register would remember that some nice person had made her feel happy.

I only hoped I had many more moments to enjoy Mom's company.

cﾟﾟ

It was hard to remember how competent Mom used to be before her Alzheimer's. At the height of her professional career, Mom ran a large synagogue as its Executive Director. She had obviously had the skills to do so. Even in her role of grandmother, she had chosen to engage her grandkids with hands-on fun, including her infamous squirt-gun baths and the telling of elaborate bedtime stories.

I had learned, though, that Alzheimer's often started presenting itself years before the actual diagnosis was made. Scientists have learned that the loss of smell can often presage the onset of Alzheimer's.[29]

As part of her diagnosis, Mom was tested by a gerontologist with the clock-drawing test, a tool that is used to screen for signs of neurological problems. The individual is asked to draw a clock face, meaning the hours one through twelve in their customary positions within a circle, then add the minute and hour hands to a specific requested time, often eleven-ten. The simple scoring method consists of giving a point if the clock is completed accurately and no points if the clock is completed inaccurately. The conclusion is if a normal clock is drawn, it indicates the absence of dementia; an abnormally drawn clock is cause for further evaluation.

Most recently, Mom was tested in March 2017 by her gerontologist to assess her abilities. She could not draw a clock correctly. She couldn't even remember the city in which she lived or the current year. She was angry at being tested and, as if she knew that much depended on it, fearful at her inability to answer. Her condition had obviously deteriorated.

---

[29] "Episodic Memory of Odors Stratifies Alzheimer Biomarkers in Normal Elderly," Albers, Alefiya Dhilla, Phd, et al., Annals of Neurology, Vol. 80, No. 6, December 2016, pp. 846-857.

For me, finding Mom's last cookbook made me realize how tenuous her skills had become.

We were cleaning up the storage area in my parent's laundry room when a stained, ripped book slid in a cloud of dust from the top shelf above the washing machine and literally fell into my hands. "What's this?" I wondered. The book's binding was missing, and the back cover was hanging by a thread. With great curiosity, I opened the front cover to find Mom's hand-written recipe for "Sesame Green Beans" taped on the inside. This was followed by a few pages of ads and then the title page: *Florence Greenberg's Jewish Cookery Book,* Sixth Edition.[30] I had never seen this book in my life. I thought Mom had given me all of her cookbooks. How had this one escaped my notice?

First published in 1947, Greenberg's cookbook grew out of a post-World War II need to be thrifty in all things, especially food. Greenberg's husband, Leopold, was publisher of the British Jewish newspaper, *The Jewish Chronicle*, on which Greenberg served as "cookery editor." She packed her cookbook with no-nonsense, comprehensive recipes, many of which were not particularly Jewish in flavor; the tenets of keeping kosher, the system by which religious Jews separate the cooking of meat and milk, takes up little space, and "Traditional Jewish Dishes" are relegated to a specific chapter. And yet, this cookbook—reprinted thriteen times between 1947 and 1977[31]—was an essential part of most British Jewish households.

The importance of the book lay beyond what was printed in it, for stuffed between the pages I found loose

---

[30] Greenberg, Florence, *Florence Greenberg's Jewish Cookery Book,* Sixth Edition (Jewish Chronicle Publications, London, 1958).
[31] Russell, Polly, "The History Cook: Jewish Cookery by Florence Greenberg," *Financial Times,* August 15, 2014.

pieces of paper. Some were filled with doodles and names, phone numbers, and addresses from Mom's life prior to moving to Israel. Others held recipes or full menus for long-forgotten meals. There were also notes that were obviously written after Mom's move to Israel. I could barely read these. When had her handwriting become so bad?

Looking through the cookbook, I was reminded of Drora's story about collecting her mother's things when she moved her mom to an assisted living facility. Aliza's Alzheimer's was noticeable. She barely spoke, even to her daughter, as if afraid that her inability to understand conversations would be discovered. Among her possessions was an address book, and inside the front cover, Aliza had written many iterations of the current year and below it her birth year. Apparently she was trying desperately to determine how old she was by subtracting one from the other. The handwriting had deteriorated so much that it was barely decipherable.

Florence Greenberg's Jewish Cookery Book was bursting with hundreds of recipes and many strange cooking tips, such as: "There is no need to waste a single crust of stale bread, for there are endless ways in which it can be used," or "Experience will soon teach you to gauge the heat of the oven by putting the hand in for a moment. Beginners can test by putting a piece of white paper on a shelf. If it turns dark brown in 4 or 5 minutes—hot oven. If it turns light brown—moderately hot oven. If it turns light yellow—moderate oven."

The book was replete with funny-sounding recipes like "Carrot Candy," "Sand Cake," "Ox Tongue with Caper Sauce," "Pickled Damsons" (referring to damson plums—I didn't know what a damson was either!), and a whole chapter on "Invalid Cookery," which, as I eventually figured out, meant cooking for sick people.

I enjoyed looking through the cookbook, sensing its damaged past and Mom's connection to it. I was especially interested in the recipes Mom had chosen to add in her own handwriting and tape inside the book. After spending several hours with Florence Greenberg, I wasn't sure what to do with the cookbook. While I didn't think I'd use it much, I put a big rubber band around it to keep it together and gave it a place on my shelf. If it had served Mom well, it deserved to be kept for further contemplation.

I delighted in putting to use some of Florence Greenberg's practical suggestions. And I immediately adopted as my own Mom's recipe for sesame green beans.

Sesame Green Beans

I found this recipe written in Mom's handwriting taped to the inside cover of Florence Greenberg's cookbook. I'm not sure how long it had been there or if Mom had ever made these for me, but I was very happy to add her recipe to my repertoire. This has become one of our all-time favorite ways to eat green beans. It is simple to prepare and can be eaten hot or cold. I even shared it with members of my synagogue in a communal cookbook that came out in 2014. To toast sesame seeds, pour your seeds into a frying pan over a high flame and, using the handle of the pan, gently swish the seeds around as they brown. You'll end up with multi-hued seeds ranging from dark brown to light brown. This takes about ten minutes.

2 Tbsp sesame oil
1 Tbsp canola oil
4 to 5 garlic cloves, crushed
1 28 oz / 800 gr bag frozen green beans, uncut
¼ cup soy sauce
⅛ cup toasted sesame seeds

Directions:
In a large sauce pan, sauté garlic in oil. Add frozen green beans and cook until defrosted, stirring occasionally. Add soy sauce and sesame seeds. Stir and simmer for ten minutes. Serve warm or cold.

Marilyn's Stuffing

Putting Florence Greenberg's advice into practice, here's a savory stuffing recipe that will use up every stale bread crumb in your house. We don't often make turkey in Israel, but when we do, we use my mother-in-law's stuffing recipe. I've learned many things from Marilyn, including the art of never staying still.

2 Tbsp olive oil
3 cloves garlic, crushed
1 large onion, chopped
4 to 5 stalks celery, chopped
2 red peppers, chopped
1 sliced bread loaf
½ cup fresh dill
2 tsp dried parsley
Salt and pepper to taste
2 eggs
1 ½ -2 cups water

Directions:
Lay slices of bread on a large baking pan and toast in oven on 420 degrees F / 210 degrees C until they begin to brown. Flip bread slices and toast the second side. Remove from oven and cool. In a frying pan, sauté garlic and onion. Add vegetables, dill, and spices. Cook until vegetables are soft. In a large bowl, break the toasted bread into chunks. Stir in vegetable mixture. Mix together water and eggs then pour over bread and vegetables until coated. Stuff mixture into the cavity of the turkey or chicken and cook according to the bird's weight. Place remaining stuffing in a baking dish and bake at 350 degrees F / 180 degrees C until the top starts to brown.

Plum Pie

Israel grows a variety of plums, including the Hanita that looks a lot like the Damson plum. Mom loves plums; and this is one of our favorite summer recipes.

¾ cup plus 2 Tbsp canola oil
½ cup sugar
2 eggs
2½ cups flour
12 purple plums, halved and pitted (or enough to cover the crust)
3 Tbsp lemon juice

Topping:
¼ cup canola oil
¾ cup sugar
3 Tbsp flour
2 tsp cinnamon

Directions:
Preheat oven to 350 degrees F / 180 degrees C. Beat sugar, oil and eggs in a bowl. Add flour to mixture and form a dough. Pat into a greased nine-inch / twenty-three-cm pie pan. Layer plum halves skin side up on dough. In another bowl, combine topping ingredients. You may want to double the topping. Sprinkle plums with lemon juice and dot topping over plum halves. Bake for thirty minutes.

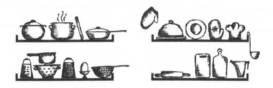

Alzheimer's Lens

My mother's mother died in the winter
of her years. All that she left us
save for photos and wrinkled bits of paper—
and her precious Scrabble board—
was a large-handled magnifying glass
still wrapped in its original packaging.

My mother did not remember.
And I, her oldest granddaughter,
magnified my grief to compensate.

Chapter 14

The Final Chapter

I am sorry to call you this early," the voice explained on the phone, "but we can't reach your father, Jack. I'm calling from Nofei Hasharon Nursing Home where we've just pronounced the death of your grandmother Millie Silverstein."

My Booba died at the age of 101 in January 2017. Despite her age, I was not prepared to hear this news. With my heart racing and my knees buckling, I tried to carry on the conversation about the bureaucratic procedures involved in finalizing a death, but it was too much for me. I hung up the phone and burst into tears.

My grandmother was such a fixture in my life that it was impossible for me to contemplate her absence. How many people are fortunate enough to have an adult relationship with their grandparents? How many of us are able to carry that relationship through to our children and grandchildren? One of the last times we saw Booba, we introduced her to her great-great-grandchild. The minute she saw baby Roi, she was transformed, actively cooing and calling to him, engaging with him in smiles and sounds. What a difference from the nearly comatose existence she led. Booba had been confined to a wheelchair due to a fracture in her hip from a fall in 2011 that had never healed. Her eyesight, bad when I was a kid, was almost non-existent, and her hearing, too, was also almost gone.

I reached Daddy by phone, then made the difficult calls to my aunt and cousins in London, my brother in California, my children, and my husband Jeff who was attending a conference in New Jersey. Jewish tradition requires the burial to occur as soon as possible after death; it was agreed that we would delay the funeral for two days until my Auntie Barbara arrived.

And what would we tell Mom? Mom visited Booba two or three times each week. She doted on her mother, often holding her hand or singing to her. On the other hand, Mom didn't always remember my grandmother was wheelchair bound or 100-plus-years-old. Sometimes, Mom was sure her mother was out shopping. Would she understand that her mother had died?

What about the traditional *shiva*? This was a little more complicated. *Shiva* is the week-long mourning period for first-degree relatives—father, mother, son, daughter, brother, sister, and spouse—who, immediately after the burial, sit in either their home or the home of the deceased and accept condolences from friends and relatives who wish to share in their sorrows. How long would Auntie Barbara stay in Israel? Could Mom be in a situation where she was constantly reminded of her mother's death? Did she understand the concept of mourning?

I finally managed to catch a mid-morning train to Netanya. By the time I arrived, though she had broken down in tears when she was told, Mom had forgotten all about her mother's death.

We'd been making arrangements all day. Each time we mentioned the word "funeral," Mom asked who had died. She wanted to know why we were whispering and why she wasn't included in the conversations. I showed her a photo of her sister Barbara and told her that Barbara was coming to visit. But it didn't really sink in.

We decided that Mom would come to the funeral, and then, as is traditional, she and her sister would sit *shiva* for a short period of time until Barbara returned to England. Mom would not sit for the full week. How could she if she couldn't even hold in her mind the painful truth of losing her mother.

Daddy and I decided that Mom had the right to know about her mother's death. She had the right to grieve and feel loss—as we all do—as she was still capable of feeling. If she wanted to know details, I'd tell her.

Do I recommend informing all Alzheimer's patients about a death or tragedy that may affect them adversely? The decision depends on the state of the individual when such an event occurs. And it depends on how they are told—with kindness, in a safe place, perhaps holding hands and crying together. There is no right or wrong choice, just one that may be more painful than another.

My dad got it right when he said about my grandmother: "Millie was someone who left an indelible mark on all those who met her and we will never see her like again."

It wasn't a tragic loss. My grandmother's quality of life had shrunk considerably. She was not really lucid. She needed assistance for every aspect of her daily tasks. My brother Simon had mentally said his goodbyes about seven years earlier when Booba had had so many mini strokes that her mind had been lost to dementia, her hands had curled in and her functionality diminished considerably; she could no longer beat him or even play at

Scrabble, her prowess as the family champion finally over.

It was a loss nonetheless, made complicated by Mom's inability to mourn. No matter what we did, Alzheimer's was always with us, shadowing us and throwing darkness on our lives. It made it more difficult to mourn, to give in to our sadness, because Mom reacted to our emotions. To keep her calm and cheerful, we had to be calm and cheerful.

At the funeral, Mom cycled through several emotions. At one point, as she was walking to the gravesite, she told my aunt Barbara that she had forgotten to tell her mother where she was. I sucked in my breath over that one. Then she repeatedly told me it was a waste of her time to be there.

So, too, at the *shiva* that we held in my parent's apartment. Mom listened to all the stories we told about Booba then asked if the person we were speaking about was still alive. When someone told her no, she angrily yelled out, "My mother is not dead!"

On the advice of Mom's caregiver Rachel, we started talking about the death of our "friend." It was easier to shield Mom that way from the repeated discovery of her mother's passing.

My grandmother was a big presence in my life. I was her first grandchild born a day before her 50th birthday. She apparently made it her mission to bless me by superstitiously holding her thumb between her fingers—*holting a farge* she called it—and telling everyone how ugly I was, the opposite of what she truly felt. Her large, uncompromising personality accompanied me as I grew and developed. Those early years were filled with frustration at the way she embarrassed me with her outspoken criticisms, her bossy nature, and the all-encompassing strength of her own convictions.

All that changed when, during college, I spent a month with my grandparents in their Netanya apartment—my grandfather Hilly was still alive then. I learned to appreciate their give-and-take, their dedication to friends, their activism and volunteerism. I also accepted that though we were related, I was not responsible for their crazy antics.

Booba would unabashedly tell me how famous she was in Netanya, how everyone knew her because she used to attend Israeli folk dances every Saturday night in the town square (while Hilly sat on the sidelines and played his drum).

She boasted about how well she danced. "Yeah, right," I would think to myself. And then one day, walking in the streets of the city, a stranger came up to us and said, "Oh, I know you! You're that wonderful dancer in the square!"

She once stopped a pick-pocket with her umbrella.

I will always remember her telling me about the time she forgot to put on her "knickers" before she went out and how the strong wind kept blowing her skirt and exposing her nether parts.

Or the time we were stuck in a small, hot car in the middle of a safari in England and she took off her shirt to cool down. Sitting in the back seat with her four grandchildren, her pointy white bra shone like a beacon. She was more interesting than any wild animal to the passengers in the bus that pulled up next to us. And I, being twelve, wanted to hide in shame.

Mom has often demanded to "go home" to her parents when evening descends. Strangely, though, she has never once requested that we visit Booba. It is as if her mother has ceased to exist for her. Mom's one primary comfort is my dad. No one can replace him.

As for my grandmother, if Mom asks, I've already decided to tell her that Booba is out shopping for all eternity.

 ⌒⌒⌒

Learning how to make something out of very little was a skill that Mom inherited from her mother and passed on to me through her cooking. I can recall the nights when I stood on my chair in the kitchen looking out the window past the yellow curtains, past the large pink dogwood that bloomed in our yard, past the end of the empty driveway to the curved curb along the quiet road where I waited for signs of Daddy's return. The minute I saw his car round the corner at the intersection near our house, I'd jump down and announce for all to hear that it was time for dinner.

Daddy would saunter in, put down his bag, and yell out, "Where's my dinner?"

"Where'd you leave it?" we'd all shout back.

The meals Mom patched together from leftovers were legendary in our house. We called them, Leftovers Supreme. She'd bring to the table a pan brimming with chicken or beef cut into small pieces and sautéed with as many vegetables as would fit. She'd add onion and peppers, maybe leftover green beans or cauliflower. If she had only meat remaining, she'd use all fresh vegetables to make a colorful dish, often adding broccoli, peas, or carrots. She'd add soy sauce or tomato paste, or, if we were lucky, unused gravy to create a delectable sauce.

It didn't matter what she put in. What mattered was her ability to create something out of nothing. This was part of our family's living within its means, the goal of not wasting anything. In this age of plenty, it's hard to remember that my parents grew up in post WWII London where money was tight. Their childhood, lived in the noisy, busy streets of the East End, was nothing like my privileged upbringing in the suburbs of middle-class America.

I too, have internalized this lesson. In Israel, we make everything from scratch. When I first moved here, instant cake mixes were unheard of. If you wanted cake, you made it the old fashioned way. Today, with so many conveniently packaged meals and sauces and instant dinners in the freezer section of every grocery store, it is important for me to purchase wisely and cook within my budget. In this country, fast food is more expensive than a slow-cooked home-made meal: a Big Mac meal at McDonald's costs the equivalent of $9.50 in New Israeli Shekels and a Double Mac Royal more than $14.00. I save our leftovers in all-sized containers, sighing happily when another one is put empty into the sink.

I can't say there hasn't been grumbling from my kids when dinner appears on the table as a changed version of yesterday's fare. I hope, though, that the lesson of waste not, want not is one they take to heart in their own future homes.

As when I was growing up, every time we make Mom's "Leftovers Supreme," it turns out different. It's all in the quality of what you've got to put in it. And the amount of love you add. Sort of like our lives.

Leftovers Supreme

Here are general instructions for making this dish. Be creative. Try strange combinations and wow yourself with how well they combine. Or remember not to repeat them if they don't. Recently I used a ¼ cabbage sliced thin, some rather limp celery, a large over-ripe tomato, two carrots, an abandoned half pepper, 1½ Tbsp salsa (that's all that was left), and chickpeas, and added it to four leftover chicken pieces cut into strips. Voila! Serve with rice or even tortillas.

Directions:

Fry some garlic and onion then add your choice of vegetables. Cook about ten minutes on a medium flame until vegetables are cooked through. Toss in about one pre-cooked chicken piece per person deboned and cut into strips. Lower flame and simmer for another ten minutes. Add salt and pepper to taste.

Here's where it gets interesting. To add flavor to your dish, you may want to use either cumin or soy sauce, a cup of crushed tomatoes, or sweet and sour chili sauce. The sky's the limit.

Questions my Mother Asked,
Answers my Father Gave Her

Where were you last night?
I was here, with you,
though you thought I was your father.
Where were you last night?
Out dancing with my imaginary lover
who never forgets my name.

Where are the children?
They are grown with children of their own.
They live in their own homes.
Where are the children?
They are waiting in the silken sky
for your goodnight kisses.

Do you want a cup of tea?
Not now. I'm busy. You made some an hour ago.
Do you want a cup of tea?
I want many things. I want to stand with you
under the canopy and never look forward.

How many children did I give birth to?
You cradled them both in your arms,
raised them to adulthood.
How many children did I give birth to?
Daughter earth is calling. Go gently to her.

Where are my keys?
I told you. Check the back pocket of your bag.
Where are my keys?
We are locked inside this room together.

Is it time yet?
We have plenty of time.
Is it time yet?
Yes, it is time.

after Mark Strand

AFTERWORD

Mom doesn't know about this book. And I can't tell her. Though she doesn't have the ability to read much anymore, if she did read it, she'd be angry and insulted and insist there's nothing wrong with her. On the other hand, she might forget that I'd told her about it and then accuse me of intentionally keeping her in the dark.

It's hard to hide such an intimate project from someone I love. It makes me feel dishonest—I *am* intentionally keeping her in the dark.

If I were writing an advice column about Alzheimer's, I'd say learn from my mistakes. I've made plenty in taking care of Mom, and I figure I'll be making a lot more in the future. I still smart at the time Daddy took Mom to the bathroom at a restaurant where we were eating lunch and I missed her return. I guess Mom came out before him and made her way to the outside tables. I was sitting right where she'd left me, but she didn't see me. And I, playing with my phone, didn't see her either. It must have been a few minutes before Daddy came out and found her pacing the restaurant in utter fear. She even shouted at me.

"How dare you move away when I'm looking for you!" she yelled.

It took another few minutes to pacify her and apologize for my serious lack of attention.

✺✺✺

I grew up singing John Prine's song "Dear Abby,"[32] a humorous look at the kinds of people who write to advice columnists. Be satisfied with who you are and what

---

[32] Prine, John, "Dear Abby," *Sweet Revenge.* Atlantic Records, 1973.

you have, the song implies. Of course, Calvin of *Calvin and Hobbes* comics fame, takes a different perspective. His suggestion: all the whiny people of the world should suck it up and stop whining.[33] Here's some advice I've gleaned these past few years. I offer it in the hopes it will help you if you are going through something similar.

Each individual with Alzheimer's is unique, so there's no telling if what works for my mom will work for you. In fact, sometimes, what works one day with Mom won't work the next. Bottom line: be creative. This is a by-the-seat-of-your-pants operation.

Probe gently. What kind of mood is Mom in today? Is she hostile and guarded about her independence? Will she accept my help? It is better to make suggestions than to ask questions. Not, "Would you like my help?" but "Can I adjust the water temperature in the shower for you?" If you are rebuffed, keep trying. She needs you; she just doesn't realize it and can't express it.

Use improv. If Mom is talking about how someone had something that they had to deliver but it went astray and what should she do and does she need money and is this the letter (holding up her nightgown) that she needs, counter with your own illogical answer. "Oh, yes, she found the right monkeys to give it to. They were very happy to drink tea and visit the queen." Mom will eventually realize you're joking with her, and hopefully start to laugh. (My husband Jeff is a pro at this.)

Live in the now. The power of the present allows Mom to laugh and sing and enjoy life fully without the pressure of having to remember the past or plan for the future.

Stay calm. My mood affects everyone around me,

---

[33] Watterson, Bill, "Newspaper Advice Columnist," Calvin & Hobbes, April 3, 1992

sometimes inadvertently. If I'm a little tired or even taciturn, Mom will pick up on that. And if something strange happens, like she starts coating her arms and chest with deodorant or brushes toothpaste into her hair, if you yell at her to stop, she may startle or become defensive. ("I know what I'm doing. Don't tell me what I can do!") Instead, swallow your incredulity and hand her a towel or hop like rabbits to the bathroom.

Change the way you speak. Alzheimer's sufferers don't remember things. It is pointless to ask, "Do you remember…" It places needless stress on Mom.

Throw out your anger. Anger is a counter-productive emotion at the best of times. How much more so when you are dealing with an Alzheimer's patient. Mom does not act out of malice; she simply can't help herself. It makes Mom extra tense and irrational when we are angry with her, which in turn prompts her own angry, venomous reactions.

Let them talk. I don't have to correct Mom's version of reality. I don't have to respond to every half-baked statement. If Mom says her food is tasteless or she's worried that she hasn't seen her parents in a long time, or she has things to do and must get home, say nothing. If Mom introduces me as her sister or cousin, let it slide. At least I know she still values me as a close relative.

When in doubt, sing. We have a song for brushing teeth and washing hair, a song for putting on Mom's medicinal patch, walking songs, eating songs, sleeping songs, songs for good moods, silly songs, and old favorites. Tap into their early memories and sing away. It doesn't matter if you can't carry a tune. Definitely learn the words to "I've got a lovely bunch of coconuts."[34]

---

[34] A novelty song composed in 1944 by Fred Heatherton, the song was a top-ten hit in the U.S. in 1950

Always know where they are. It happens gradually, their inability to function, their loss of time, of reality. You'll have to decide for yourself when you can no longer trust them to be on their own. At that point, make sure someone is with them at all times. Even if it is sitting amiably and quietly in the living room listening to music, they should not be alone. Don't let them out of your sight: they can do foolish things, like putting on five pair of underwear or cutting an electrical cord with scissors to turn off the light. Really. This is particularly daunting but necessary.

Shield them as much as possible. Stay away from noisy environments. Keep a watchful eye. Always be where she can find you. Avoid upsetting topics, like the death of a loved one.

Be prepared. Okay, you can't really be prepared, but you can train yourself to realize that each day will bring its own challenges, burdens, and goals. When I took care of Mom for two weeks on my own, I felt this crazy sinking feeling each time Mom stood in her living room and told me she had to go home. By the third or fourth time it happened, my sense of disbelief gave way to a sort of practicality in helping her find her way "home."

Accept their non-normative behavior. This is a hard one. It really depends on whether you can accept what they're doing. Should I let Mom sleep in her clothes? What about wearing her glasses to bed? How about putting on a winter coat in the middle of summer? Singing loudly in public? Wearing mismatched shoes? Refusing to wash her hair? Some of these behaviors resolve themselves as Mom's abilities falter and she relies on a caregiver to make her food or choose her clothes. Others you just might have to put up with until you find a solution.

Use their memory loss. This might sound cruel, but if you know they won't remember what you asked or requested five minutes ago, ask again in another minute. Maybe this time Mom will acquiesce and take off her glasses or swallow her pills. You can show her the same movie or sing the same songs over and over and she'll never get bored.

Pay attention. Yes, I'd rather be on my phone, or furthering my own agenda, but if I'm not focused, not only will I miss Mom's amazing statements ("That man is wearing sleeves on his knees.") but she'll also manage to do something silly like fill the frying pan with water so she can have a drink.

Don't take it personally. When she's angry, Mom may lash out. She calls me horrible names and employs curse words liberally. She uses words I never knew were in her vocabulary. It's not personal. Really. These are imbalanced brain chemicals and tangles speaking. Deep down she still loves me, and when her anger has ebbed, she'll let me know.

Take time for yourself. Oh, this is a big one. There is a reason people hire non-family members to care for their loved ones. We are so close, so connected, that it is hard to separate our own needs from the people we love most. Make sure you have good, responsible individuals backing you up and giving you down time from caregiving. When you have rest and distance, you are a better you.

Be their active memory. Play games, sing songs, show photos of kids and grandchildren, watch old movies, read poetry. Carry within you the precious moments that make up a lifetime of blessings.

When my dad came back from his September trip to the US, he was relaxed from his long break. Mom was already asleep. We talked late into the night about caring for her, how hard it was and what we could do better. When Mom woke up the next morning and saw him lying beside her, she didn't even realize he'd been away. I'd spent two weeks keeping her calm in his absence—because his absence made her unbalanced—and it was all wiped away in a single instant. How's that for gratitude?

During the late stages of this book's publication, my parents moved from Netanya to Beer Sheva to be near me. Mom's condition dramatically declined and we were forced to make the excruciating decision to institutionalize her. The care Mom receives in her memory care facility is excellent, and as the center is just ten minutes from our house, Daddy and I endeavor to visit her every day. Seeing her now makes me realize how blessed we were these past eight years to find joy in our interactions and to have had such surprising and relative stability in her condition. Mom's cognitive skills will continue to decline, along with her physical capabilities. I pray we have the strength to accompany her on her difficult journey with dignity and honor, wherever it may lead.

Whatever you do, however you approach this illness, be it your spouse or parent who is affected, give them as much love as you can even when they've forgotten who you are. Do it for them. Do it for yourself.

One meal at a time.

APPENDIX

A Guide to Alzheimer's Information and Support

As a child of someone with Alzheimer's, I am constantly on edge about my mild forgetfulness. I become dismayed when I lose words that are on the tip of my tongue. It is as if a curtain descends in my brain and the word or even the name of the person standing next to me—how embarrassing—is reduced to a fuzzy amorphousness that I can no longer articulate. When the words flood back into my mind, I am instantly grateful.

We think of losing words as a precursor to getting Alzheimer's. It is certainly one of the hallmarks of this vicious disease but unfortunately not the only one. Some studies note the loss of smell as a primary indicator of the disease.[35] Others are now labeling Alzheimer's as a third type of diabetes.[36] Many people profess to know a cure. Sadly, there isn't one yet.

It is important to know what Alzheimer's is and what Alzheimer's isn't. What signs should I look for? How will I know? And if it leaves me unscarred until my older age, are there things I can do to forestall it?

Printed here are two articles that describe the signs of Alzheimer's versus the signs of regular aging. I've also compiled several websites that I found helpful in my learning process. And, lastly, a list of books that I read,

---

[35] Brazier, Yvette, "Decreased Sense of Smell May Indicate Early Dementia," *Medical News Today,* November 16, 2015.

[36] "Alzheimer's Disease Is Type 3 Diabetes–Evidence Reviewed," Suzanne M. de la Monte, MD, MPH, and Jack R. Wands, MD, Journal of Diabetes Science and Technology, November 2008; 2(6): 1101–1113

including novels that I read expressly for pleasure. I hope you find them helpful, too.

As an added bonus, I have included a list of "Essential Tools for Cooking." This was compiled as part of the original concept behind this cookbook, called, *The Man's Emergency Cookbook.* If you've recently taken up cooking, I hope this list and the accompanying tips help you on your journey

Ten Early Signs and Symptoms of Alzheimer's[37]

1. *Memory loss that disrupts daily life.* One of the most common signs of Alzheimer's, especially in the early stages, is forgetting recently learned information or asking for the same information over and over.

2. *Challenges in planning or solving problems.* Some people may experience changes in their ability to develop and follow a plan, or work with numbers. They may have difficulty concentrating and take much longer to do things than they did before.

3. *Difficulty completing familiar tasks at home, at work or at leisure.* People with Alzheimer's often find it hard to complete daily tasks like driving to a familiar location, managing a budget at work or remembering the rules of a favorite game.

4. *Confusion with time or place.* People with Alzheimer's can lose track of dates, seasons, and the passage of time. Sometimes they may forget where they are or how they got there.

5. *Trouble understanding visual images and spatial relationships.* For some people, vision problems are a sign of Alzheimer's. They may have difficulty reading, judging distance, and determining color or contrast. They may not recognize their own reflection.

---

[37] Copyright 2009, Alzheimer's Association. All rights reserved. Reprinted with permission.

6. *New problems with words in speaking or writing.* People with Alzheimer's may have trouble following or joining a conversation. They may stop in the middle of a conversation and have no idea how to continue, or they may repeat themselves.

7. *Misplacing things and losing the ability to retrace steps.* A person with Alzheimer's disease may put things in unusual places. They may lose things and be unable to find them again. Sometimes, they may accuse others of stealing.

8. *Decreased or poor judgment.* People with Alzheimer's may experience changes in judgment or decision making. They may pay less attention to grooming or keeping themselves clean.

9. *Withdrawal from work or social activities.* A person with Alzheimer's may start to remove themselves from hobbies, social activities, work projects, or sports. They may also avoid being social because of the changes they have experienced.

10. *Changes in mood and personality.* The mood and personalities of people with Alzheimer's can become confused, suspicious, depressed, fearful, or anxious. They may be easily upset at home, at work, with friends or in places where they are out of their comfort zone.

This is an official check list of the Alzheimer's Association. For more information, go to the alz.org website.

12 Signs You Probably Don't Have Alzheimer's

There's less to worry about than you think.[38]

Are you worried that you might have Alzheimer's or another form of dementia? Many people are a bit over-worried. Watching a family member with dementia decline is enough to make anyone secretly fear his or her own occasional memory lapses or confused moments.

It's worth emphasizing the flip side to those who are in midlife and coping with work and sandwich-generation demands. The statistical odds indicate that you're probably okay. I don't say that to make light of Alzheimer's disease or the horrible fact that early-onset Alzheimer's cases are on the rise. And I would urge anybody nagged by suspicions to get them checked out pronto.

But when you're under a lot of strain, other factors can also play with your mind, such as moving too fast, not getting enough sleep, depression or plain old worry. The majority of people over age fifty—even over sixty, seventy, or eighty—don't have dementia.

So if it makes you feel any better, here are twelve signs that generally don't indicate Alzheimer's:

* Forgetting a new acquaintance's name. Everybody does it.

* Forgetting an old acquaintance's name. It's more embarrassing, but everybody does this, too.

* Remembering in the middle of the night that you forgot to put out tomorrow's trash for pick-up. The fact that you eventually remembered is positive.

* You caught another mistake when balancing your checkbook. Balancing a checkbook is a complicated task;

---

[38] Paula Spencer Scott, Caring.com Senior Editor. Reprinted with permission.

that you can do most of it flawlessly is a good sign. And slipshod math is common.

* You can't remember where you parked the car. Unless you always park in the same spot and then forget, occasionally blanking is no big deal, especially in vast lots at a shopping center, hospital or mall. Possible problem: If you have to write down where you park each and every time.

* Feeling too blah to attend book group, an activity you usually love. Losing interest in hobbies or a social life is a hallmark of the disease. But wanting to chill alone every so often is, well, *human*. Take care not to make it a habit; isolating yourself socially is also a red flag for depression.

* Losing your sunglasses—again. To misplace is human. To finally find the sunglasses in the refrigerator or the trash, on the other hand, is possible Alzheimer's.

* Your partner elbows you at a party and says, "Oh please, don't tell that story again." Over the years, couples often build up a trove of anecdotes (how we met, the time we sat next to a movie star on a plane, how we bought our house for a song, the day we learned our son was a genius). Such tales and jokes are often ignited by certain social cues. Knowing you're doing this is different from hearing, "But you just told that story five minutes ago"—and not remembering doing so.

* Not recognizing your own reflection for a second after a new haircut or new glasses. Your brain's still absorbing the new look. More worrisome: still thinking, after a moment's pause, that the person staring back at you in the mirror is someone else.

* Forgetting an appointment, or arriving on the wrong day. Big goof, but still—blame stress, multitasking or maybe needing a better planner system. Don't

worry unless this is happening routinely, instead of once in a full blue moon.

* Feeling old and baffled because you can't figure out how to text message, set up wireless access in your house, or stream video to your TV set (though the ten-year-old kid next door can). I write from experience: Technology moves faster than many a middle-aged mind. And instructions often seem written by non-English speaking tech-heads. Keeping up with progress is different from losing ground—e.g. no longer being able to follow a recipe or tell a cell phone from a TV remote.

* Saying stuff like, "that thingamabob" or "you know, that actress who was in that movie…" Sounds like typical over-forty conversation to me. Proper words for things do tend to elude people with Alzheimer's but they improvise strangely ("ice on a stick" for popsicle," hair fork" for comb). But as for peppering your talk with "thingys" and "that's," well, for that, you're still on pretty solid ground if you can still manage to Google.

Helpful Websites

The Alzheimer's Association
One of the world's leading voluntary health organizations in Alzheimer's care, support and research.
http://www.alz.org/

Alzheimer's Australia
Providing support and advocacy for the more than 321,000 Australians living with dementia.
http://www.fightdementia.org.au

Alzheimer's Disease International
The international federation of more than 79 Alzheimer associations, representing people and nations on all continents.
www.alz.co.uk/

Alzheimer's Foundation of America
Provides optimal care and services to individuals confronting dementia, and to their caregivers and families—through member organizations dedicated to improving quality of life.
http://www.alzfdn.org/

The Alzheimer's Reading Room
To educate and empower Alzheimer's caregivers, their families, and the entire Alzheimer's community.
http://www.alzheimersreadingroom.com/

Alzheimer's Research Forum
A dynamic on-line scientific community dedicated to understanding Alzheimer's disease and related disorders. The website reports on the latest scientific findings from basic research to clinical trials, creates and maintains

public databases of essential research data and reagents, and produces discussion forums to promote debate, speed the dissemination of new ideas, and break down barriers across the numerous disciplines that can contribute to the global effort to cure Alzheimer's disease.
http://alzforum.org/

Alzheimer's Society
A membership organization, which works to improve the quality of life of people affected by dementia in England, Wales and Northern Ireland.
http://www.alzheimers.org.uk/

Dementia Advocacy and Support Network
Promotes respect and dignity for persons with dementia, provides a forum for the exchange of information, encourages support mechanisms such as local groups, counseling, and internet linkages, and advocates for services.
http://dasninternational.org/

The Mayo Clinic
A nonprofit worldwide leader in medical care, research and education for people from all walks of life.
http://www.mayoclinic.com/health/alzheimers-disease/DS00161

Melabev
Israel's pioneer service provider caring for those plagued by, and suffering from, Alzheimer's disease or dementia, along with offering appropriate services to their entire support system.
http://melabev.org/

Project We Forget

A community of support for caregivers to persons with Alzheimer's and other forms of dementia.
https://projectweforgot.com

WebMD
Provides valuable health information, tools for managing your health, and support to those who seek information.
http://www.webmd.com/alzheimers/default.htm

Books on Alzheimer's and Memory Loss

There are many books, both non-fiction and fiction, that incorporate Alzheimer's and/or dementia as their main topic. One of the most well-known is *The 36-Hour Day,* which describes in detail the difficulties and possible solutions to dealing with someone with Alzheimer's. But it was the fiction books that really caught my attention. I was surprised by how many novels used dementia as a storyline. Here are a few that you might like, too.

36-Hour Day, The, 5th Edition, Nancy L. Mace, MA, and Peter V. Rabins, MD, MPH, Baltimore, Johns Hopkins University Press, 1981

Almost Moon, The, Alice Sebold, Little Brown and Company, NY, 2002

Dear Alzheimer's: A Caregiver's Diary & Poems, Esther Altshul Helfgott, Cave Moon Press, WA, 2013

Close to Me, But Far Away: Living with Alzheimer's, Burton M. Wheeler, University of Missouri Press, Columbia, MO, 2001

Cloud Keeper, The, Liza Futerman, Tampold Publishing, 2016.

Contented Dementia: 24-Hour Wraparound Care for Lifelong Well-being, Oliver James, Vermillion, London, 2008

Elizabeth is Missing, Emma Healy, HarperCollins, NY 2014

Feeding My Mother: Comfort and Laughter in the Kitchen as my Mom Lives with Memory Loss, Jan Arden, Random House, Canada, 2017

Financial Lives of the Poets, The: A Novel, Jess Walter, Harper Perennial, 2009

Life on Planet Alz, Jack Cohen, Elders of Zion Press, 2017

Musicophilia: Tales of Music and the Brain, Oliver Sacks, Vintage Books, New York, 2007

Remind Me Who I am Again, Linda Grant, Granta, London, 1999

Still Alice, Lisa Genova, New York, Simon & Schuster, 2007

Turn of Mind, Alice LaPlante, Atlantic Monthly Press, 2011

Walking One Another Home: Moments of Grace and Possibility in the Midst of Alzheimer's, Rita Bresnahan, Ligouri Publications, Ligouri, MO, 2003

Essential Tools for Cooking

If you've never cooked before, getting started can be an intimidating process. As a new cook, you may go through several stages of experimentation, like my dad did when Mom could no longer cook for the two of them. For example, Daddy quickly understood that pasta is easy to cook, and so is fish.

Here's one of the first things to do: designate a workspace in your kitchen. Once you've done that, here are a few essential tools you should have on hand when you cook:

1. A sharp knife for chopping and slicing;
2. Measuring cups for both liquids and solids;
3. Cutting boards;
4. Oven-proof casserole dish or pan;
5. Two or three pots of different sizes for the stove-top (with lids);
6. Hand-held blender (great for soups);
7. A food processor;
8. Microwave-safe pans;
9. A spatula (for scraping bowls);
9. Oven mitts; and
10. Baking Paper.

As for me, I favor a glass measuring cup so I can place it in the microwave. And I enjoy the large, thin plastic cutting boards that are lightweight and can be picked up and carried with your chopped vegetables to easily slide them into a pot or pan. Use baking paper when possible to lessen the chore of cleaning oven pans.

The recipes in this book use the imperial measuring system. For converting measurements, use these formulas:

3 Tbsp = ¼ cup = 2 oz. = 50 grams
1 cup = 8 oz. = 200 grams

Most of the recipes are cooked or baked at 350 degrees F / 180 degrees C F / 180 degrees C F (Fahrenheit). This translates to 180 degrees C (Celsius).

One more point: Onions! Many of the recipes begin with directions to sauté onions in a pan. To "sauté" is a French term for frying in a small amount of oil (or butter or other fat). Onions are sometimes hard to work with, but we don't all have to practice cutting onions like Meryl Streep in her exceptional portrayal of Julia Child in the film *Julie & Julia* in order to become an onion maven. A good, sharp knife is the key. First, peel the onion with the knife, cutting the top and bottom clear off. This will pull part of the thin peel with it. To remove the rest, use the knife to score the onion down one side from the top. Now peel the top layer or two off the onion till you reach the part you want to use. The onion can then be sliced in rings or long thin slices, chopped, grated, minced, or anything in between.

If you find your eyes watering, run the onions under water before cutting to reduce the effect. Some people say that if you stick out your tongue or hold a spoon in your mouth while you chop an onion, it will prevent your eyes from watering. I'm not sure about that.

Recipes Index

Alzheimer's Index

Credits

"Balance," from *Heroes in Disguise* by Linda Pastan. Copyright © 1991 by Linda Pastan. Used by permission of W.W. Norton & Company, Inc. (print) and by permission of Linda Pastan in care of the Jean V. Naggar Literary Agency, Inc. (ebook).

"In the Beginning," includes phrases from *Close to Me, But Far Away: Living with Alzheimer's* by Burton M. Wheeler (Columbia: University of Missouri Press, 2001). Used with permission of the University of Missouri Press.

"Brain Tangles" appeared in *The Barefoot Review,* Winter 2013

"Alzheimer's Pantoum" appeared in *The Barefoot Review,* Winter 2013

"Recipe for a Small Star" appeared in a different version in *The Barefoot Review,* Winter 2013

"Promises," in an earlier version, was awarded 2nd place in the 2012 JewishStoryWriting.com Summer! competition.

"Questions my Mother Asked, Answers my Father Gave Her" won the annual 2013 Reuben Rose Poetry competition.

"Frog in My Throat," appeared in *Red Wolf Journal,* Issue 12, Fall/Winter 2017/2018

About the Author

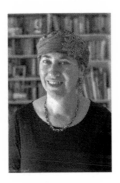

Miriam Green is a twenty-seven-year resident of Beer Sheva, Israel, the mother of three children, and grandmother of one. She lives with her husband, Jeff, two cats, and a snake named Popcorn. She blogs weekly on her website at thelostkitchen.org, chronicling her mother's Alzheimer's.

57555780R00164

Made in the USA
Columbia, SC
11 May 2019